MAYO CLINIC

GUIDE TO BETTER VISION

Sophie J. Bakri, M.D.

Medical Editor-in-Chief

Mayo Clinic
Rochester, Minnesota

Editorial staff

Medical Editor-in-Chief
Sophie J. Bakri, M.D.

Managing Editor
Kevin Kaufman

Publisher
Sara Gilliland

Editor-in-Chief, Books and Newsletters
Christopher Frye

Contributing Editors and Reviewers
Paul W. Hardwig, M.D.
Amir R. Khan, M.D.
Arthur J. Sit, M.D.
Karen Wallevand

Creative Director
Daniel Brevick

Art Directors
Stewart Koski
Paul Krause

Illustration
Michael King
Kent McDaniel
Christopher Srnka

Photography
Thomas Link
Siddiqi Ray
Jay Rostvold

Research Manager
Deirdre Herman

Research Librarian
Anthony Cook

Proofreading
Miranda Attlesey
Donna Hanson

Indexing
Steve Rath

Administrative Assistants
Karen Kulzer
Beverly Steele

Mayo Clinic Guide to Better Vision provides reliable, practical, easy-to-understand information on the diagnosis, treatment and prevention of serious eye disorders and on basic eye care and safety. Much of this information comes directly from the experience of ophthalmologists, optometrists and other health care professionals at Mayo Clinic. This book is intended to supplement the advice of your personal physician, whom you should consult regarding individual medical conditions. *Mayo Clinic Guide to Better Vision* does not endorse any company or product. MAYO, MAYO CLINIC, MAYO CLINIC HEALTH SOLUTIONS and the Mayo triple-shield logo are marks of Mayo Foundation for Medical Education and Research.

Published by Mayo Clinic Health Solutions

For bulk sales to employers, member groups and health-related companies, contact Mayo Clinic Health Management Resources, 200 First St. S.W., Rochester, MN, 55905, or send an e-mail to SpecialSalesMayoBooks@Mayo.edu.

Address inquiries to Mayo Clinic Health Solutions, Permissions Department, 200 First St. S.W., Fifth Floor Centerplace Building, Rochester, MN 55905.

Stock photography from Artville and Photodisc. The individuals pictured are models, and the photos are used for illustrative purposes only. There's no correlation between the individual portrayed and the condition or subject discussed.

Library of Congress Control Number: 2007924503

Printed in Canada

First Edition

4 5 6 7 8 9 10

Preface

Your eyes are among the most complex organs in your body. They are composites of tiny, delicate parts, synchronized to process thousands of pieces of information in an instant. In a visually oriented society such as ours, you have come to depend on your eyes for many essential activities of everyday living. Yet despite their vital importance, it is too easy to take good vision for granted.

Here's something you can do to change that. *Mayo Clinic Guide to Better Vision* provides comprehensive, in-depth coverage of many eye diseases and the basics of good eye care in a practical, easy-to-understand manner. The beginning chapters focus on chronic conditions that may cause severe vision loss if left untreated. This will help you recognize the early symptoms of diseases at a time when they are generally more treatable and before severe vision loss may have occurred. This information will also help you understand the diagnostic process and make informed treatment decisions with your doctor. Later chapters in the book explain simple ways to protect and preserve your vision.

What's the best thing about *Mayo Clinic Guide to Better Vision?* It informs you of many important advances in the diagnosis and treatment of eye disease — from technology that provides doctors with detailed images of the internal structures of the eye, to new medications for conditions that previously had been considered almost untreatable. The book also discusses improved devices and techniques for correcting many common vision problems.

Above all, we hope you enjoy reading this book and that it provides you with a better understanding of what can be done to treat eye disease and improve your vision.

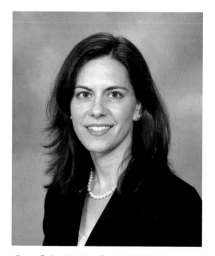

Sophie J. Bakri, M.D.
Medical Editor-in-Chief

Table of contents

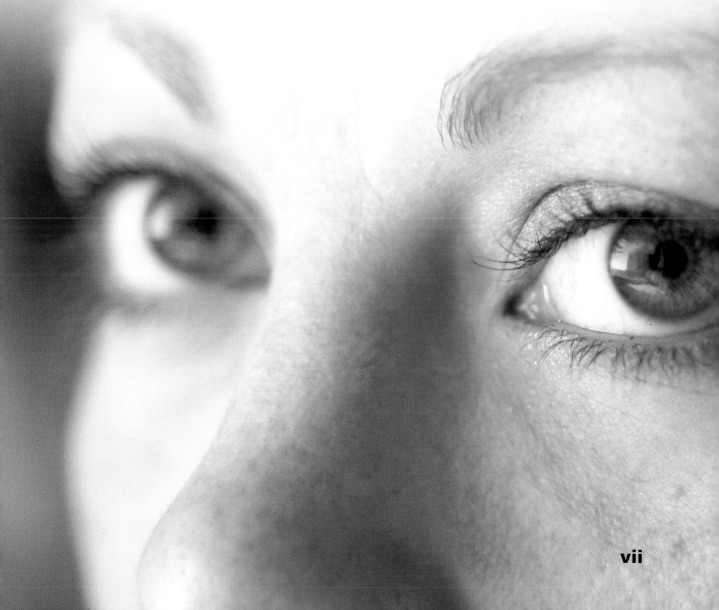

Chapter 9

Chapter 1

A look inside

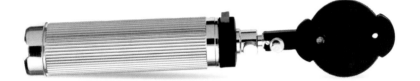

Your eyes play important roles in daily life for being such a small part of your body. Each eyeball is about an inch in diameter, just a little smaller than a table tennis ball. Vision helps you experience the shapes, colors and motions of your surroundings. It stimulates your creativity and appreciation of beauty. It alerts you to danger and the unexpected. You rely on it to explore and learn.

All five senses — sight, hearing, touch, smell and taste — are vital to your ability to function in everyday life. But sight is the sense you may have come to trust most when per-

forming many routine activities. With the help of your eyes, you read newspapers and books, write notes, balance your checkbook, drive a car, run errands, work at your job, surf the Internet, prepare meals, watch television and enjoy the theater.

On an emotional level, your vision helps define your self-image and social interactions with others. The American author Henry David Thoreau expressed it succinctly, "We are as much as we see." Given how much you depend on your eyes, it's no wonder you want to keep them as healthy as you possibly can.

Parts of the eye

People often compare the mechanisms of the eye to that of a camera, and there are certain similarities. Like a camera, each eye allows light to enter its interior through an adjustable opening at the front. An internal lens focuses the light onto a layer of light-sensitive cells at the back of the eyeball, similar to the light-sensitive film used in the camera.

This comparison, however, doesn't do your eyes justice. They have a far more complex and sophisticated function than any camera, or other piece of technology for that matter. For one thing it's a pair of eyes we're talking about, which perform together in perfect synchronization. The materials that make up the eyeball are super-flexible, resilient and lightweight.

Each eye autoregulates many rapid adjustments for brightness, focus and internal pressure. Light striking the back of the eyeball induces chemical reactions in the cells that generate electric impulses. These impulses trigger a two-way communication between the eyes and a command center in the brain. As a result of this communication, your eyes can provide sharp binocular vision and are able to follow rapid movement. All of these features give you vivid, colorful, 3-D motion pictures faster than you can blink an eye, literally.

Following is a brief description of the various structures of the eye and how they work together. Each structure plays an essential role in the healthy functioning of the eye. And each structure can be a cause of specific eye problems.

Sclera and conjunctiva

When you look in the mirror and see the white of your eye, you're looking at the sclera (SKLERE-uh) — the tough, white, leathery coating that forms the circular shape of the eyeball and protects its delicate internal structures. The sclera has a single opening at the front that allows light inside the eye.

A thin, moist, transparent membrane called the conjunctiva (kun-JUNK-ti-vuh) covers the exposed portion of the sclera. Along its edges, this tissue layer folds forward to also line the inside of your eyelids. The conjunctiva helps protect and lubricate your eye.

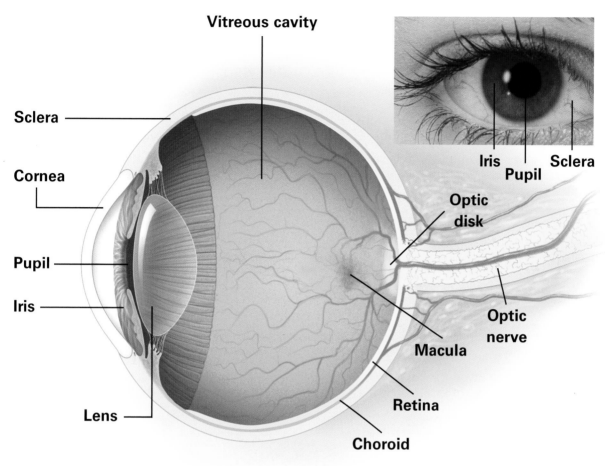

Vitreous cavity

Sclera

Cornea

Pupil

Iris

Lens

Iris
Pupil
Sclera

Optic disk

Optic nerve

Macula

Retina

Choroid

Anatomy of the eye

The complex structure of the eye is compact, measuring only about 1 inch in diameter. Yet in an instant, the eye is able to receive millions of bits of unrelated stimuli from the outside world and relay them to the visual cortex in the brain.

Cornea

The cornea is located at the front of your eye, and it covers the opening in the sclera. Comparable in shape to the crystal of a small wristwatch, it juts out from the eyeball in the form of a tiny, domed bulge.

The convex surface of the cornea bends the light entering your eye to help you focus on the object you're looking at. The eye's internal lens fine-tunes and sharpens the image.

The cornea — which is made up of several layers of tissue — also protects your eye. It's packed with sensitive nerve endings. When a tiny speck of dust hits the cornea, your brain receives the message instantly. If tears can't wash away the foreign particle, the continuing irritation prods you to locate and remove it.

Pupil

That dark spot at the center of your eye is actually a hole in the sclera — like the dark opening of a cave. This hole, called the pupil, is protected by your cornea. It's through the pupil that light passes into your eye.

Iris

Surrounding your pupil is the iris, the colored part of your eye. Its color comes from a pigment called melanin (MEL-uh-nin). The more pigment there is in your iris tissue, the darker its color. Brown eyes have a lot of pigment. Blue or green eyes have less pigment. As you get older, the color may change as your iris loses some of the pigment.

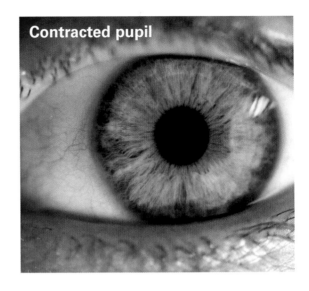

Contracted pupil

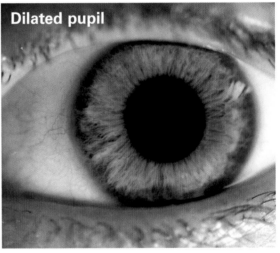

Dilated pupil

Adjustments of the iris

The iris adjusts the size of the pupil according to the amount of light. In normal light, the average pupil is open a little more than a tenth of an inch, about half the size of a pencil eraser. But its diameter can range from about six one-hundredths of an inch in bright light to about a third of an inch in low light.

The iris adds more than color to your eye. It's essentially a ring of muscle fibers that expand or contract the size of the pupil, and thereby control the amount of light that gets inside the eye. It's like adjusting blinds to control sunlight coming through a window. When the light is bright, the iris reacts quickly to reduce the size of the pupil. When the light is dim, the iris enlarges the size of the pupil.

The muscles of your iris react to more than light. Your emotions can affect the size of your pupils. Anger makes them smaller, while excitement and pleasure opens them wider. Certain drugs can open (dilate) the pupils. Doctors use dilating drugs to get a better look inside your eyes during an eye examination.

The space between the cornea and iris is called the anterior chamber. It's filled with a clear fluid called aqueous humor, which nourishes the cornea and lens, clears waste products, and plays a role in maintaining normal pressure in the eye. The aqueous humor is continuously produced in the eye, and the excess amount drains through an opening called Schlemm's canal, located in the angle where the cornea and iris meet.

Lens

Located directly behind the pupil is the lens, a clear, elliptical structure about the size and shape of an M&M'S candy. The ciliary muscles surround and support the lens. As the muscles relax or contract, the curvature of the lens changes. When an object is nearby, the muscles contract and the elastic lens becomes thicker and more curved in the middle.

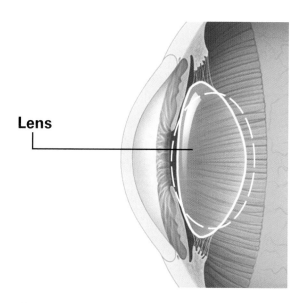

Lens

Accommodation of the lens

Changes in the shape of the lens accommodate distance vision (solid line) and close-up vision (dashed line). The thicker the lens, the more that light is refracted and the better the eye can see objects close up.

20/20 vision

It's great when an eye doctor says that you have 20/20 vision. However, that doesn't mean that you have perfect vision. It simply means that you can see objects clearly from 20 feet away — similar to what an average of people with normal sight can see clearly from 20 feet away. The term *20/20 vision* refers to your visual acuity — a measure of how sharply or clearly you can see something from a certain distance.

If you're nearsighted and have 20/50 vision, distant objects will look blurry and indistinct. In fact, they'll look so blurry that what you can see well from 20 feet away is what people with normal vision generally can see well from 50 feet away. Some people have sharper vision than 20/20. Some have 20/15 vision, or even 20/10.

There's no such thing as perfect vision. That's because many factors other than visual acuity affect your ability to see well. Even if you can see what you should from 20 feet away, your doctor will also check for other factors that can affect your vision. These include your depth perception, color vision, contrast sensitivity, peripheral vision and ability to focus on close objects.

When an object is far away, the muscles relax and the lens becomes thinner and flatter. These adjustments (accommodations) allow the lens to change its focusing power and sharpen the definition of an object at any distance. The variable focusing power of the lens fine-tunes the fixed focusing power of the cornea. As you get older, your lens loses some of its elasticity, and you may have difficulty focusing on objects that are close up.

Vitreous cavity

The vitreous cavity extends from the back of the lens to the retina. The cavity is filled with a clear, gelatinous substance called the vitreous humor, or simply, the vitreous, which accounts for about two-thirds of the volume and weight of the eye. The vitreous is about 99 percent water mixed with certain chemicals that make it a jelly-like consistency. Together with the aqueous humor, the vitreous helps maintain the shape of the eyeball and protect the internal structures.

The vitreous is clear, so light can pass through it to the retina. You may occasionally notice what look like tiny bits of string or lint darting through your vision. These are called floaters, and are condensed strands of vitreous or pigment. A sudden onset of floaters, especially when associated with flashing lights or hazy vision, can be a sign of potentially serious eye problems.

Retina

On the inside wall at the back of the eye is a thin layer of tissue called the retina. This term comes from a Latin word meaning "net." It's an apt name because your retina consists of millions of light-sensitive cells and nerve cells that capture the images focused onto them by your cornea and lens.

The cells (sometimes called photoreceptors) can be either rods or cones, which react to different wavelengths of light. Rod cells allow you to see in very dim light or off to the side while looking straight ahead (peripheral, or side, vision), but they can't distinguish colors. Cone cells distinguish color exquisitely but require more light to function. That's why it can be hard to see color in the evening or in dim light. (Hence the saying, "At night all cats are gray.")

There are about 20 rod cells for every cone cell on the retina. Cone cells are concentrated in the center of your

retina, allowing you to see the sharpest details when you're looking straight ahead at a well-lit object.

Light striking the rods and cones triggers a chemical reaction. This reaction generates electrical impulses that are relayed through the optic nerve to the visual cortex, the seeing portion of your brain. The image that your retina receives is upside-down. It's also reversed, similar to how you see a reversed image of yourself when you look in a mirror. The convex shapes

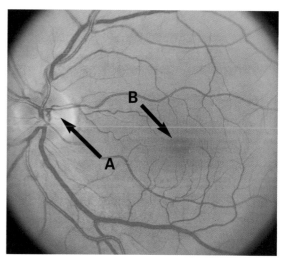

Retina

A healthy retina has an even reddish hue. The optic disk is the yellowish-orange circle with blood vessels radiating from it (arrow A). The macula is the deep red spot near the center of the retina (arrow B).

of the cornea and lens cause these effects. Your brain reinterprets this information, allowing you to see the images in their correct orientation.

The outer portion of your retina is nourished by the choroid, a layer of small arteries and veins sandwiched between the retina and the sclera. The inner retina receives its nutrition from an intricate network of retinal blood vessels. The retina and choroid are also discussed on pages 22-23.

Macula and fovea

Appearing as a dark reddish patch at the center of your retina is the macula. It's densely packed with cone cells and has only a few rod cells. The macula provides your central, or straight-ahead, vision and allows you to see fine detail when you're reading and doing other forms of close-up work. Within the macula is a small depression called the fovea (FO-vee-uh), which contains only cone cells and provides your sharpest vision.

Optic nerve

The visual information gathered by your retina is converted into electric impulses and is carried to the brain's visual cortex by a dense bundle of over 1 million nerve fibers. This communication cable between your eyes and your brain is called the optic nerve. The brain instantly decodes the impulses, coordinating signals from both eyes to produce a clear, 3-D image.

A yellowish circle that's visible on the retina indicates where the optic nerve forms at the back of the eye (see photo on page 7). This location is called the optic disk.

Muscles of the eye

Each eyeball has six muscles attached to the sclera, allowing you to move both eyes up and down and side to side. These eye muscles, which can work individually or together, allow you to track an object without necessarily having to turn your head. Your brain coordinates these movements so that both eyes move in unison when tracking an object.

Orbit

Your eyes are cradled in the orbits, which are sockets formed by a protective structure of heavy bone. This

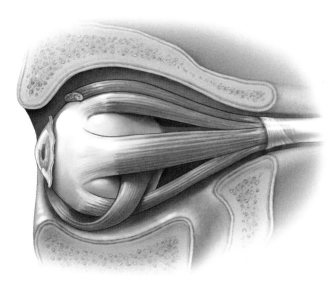

Eye socket

The orbit, or eye socket, is a cone-shaped bony cavity that protects the eye. The socket is padded with fatty tissue that allows the eye to move easily. Six muscles are in charge of eye movement: up, down, right, left and the twisting motion of the eye when you tilt your head.

structure includes the cheekbone, forehead bone, temple bone and bridge of your nose. Unlike other bones in your body, these eye protectors usually don't weaken and thin with age. Fat, muscle and other tissue cushion the eyeball within the orbit.

Upper and lower eyelids protect the front of your eyeball by blocking

debris and bright light that can damage your eyes. The eyelids also lubricate your eye with each blink. Blinking washes away dirt, pollen and other foreign particles. The lubricant, familiar to us as tears, comes from lacrimal glands located above each eye.

When something irritates your eye, such as chemical vapor from the onion you're peeling, the tear glands open up. If the tearing is slight, fluid will drain through tiny ducts within each eyelid and into your nose, taking the irritants with it. But this drainage system can't handle fully opened glands. That's when tears overflow the eyelids and run down your cheeks, such as when you're crying.

Age-related changes

Your vision typically changes as you get older. Many of these changes are primarily an annoyance and over time you learn to adjust to them. Here are some ways your eyes change with time, and how these differences affect your vision:

- Your lenses begin to cloud, causing a decrease in visual acuity. Colors become dimmer. Glare forms when light shines directly at you, causing you to avoid night driving.
- Your lenses become less elastic and lose their ability to focus on close objects — a common condition called presbyopia. Your night vision also decreases. Less elasticity may require you to continually change your reading glasses or keep a magnifying glass handy for reading small print.
- Your vitreous shrinks and fragments, which may produce bothersome floaters. You learn to ignore them, although if a sudden increase in the number of floaters occurs, you'll need to contact your eye doctor immediately.
- Tear production slows from the lacrimal glands, and the conjunctiva is no longer able to lubricate your eye and keep its surface clean. The cornea becomes drier, causing an uncomfortable, gritty sensation in the eye. Artificial-tear eyedrops may help correct the problem.

Blindness and low vision

In the United States, you're considered legally blind if the visual acuity in your best eye is 20/200 or worse even with the use of a corrective lens. People with normal vision have 20/20 vision. Blindness doesn't necessarily mean you have no sight — you may still have a limited amount of vision.

Low vision isn't the same as blindness. With low vision, you have a visual acuity of 20/70 or worse that can't be corrected with special lenses. With low vision, you may still have some functional sight but you're unable to perform many daily activities safely and you may have to depend on assistive devices.

Another common term in use is visual impairment. This is a calculation based on three independent factors: your visual acuity with corrective lenses, any loss of peripheral vision and any double vision. The score for visual impairment ranges from 0 percent to 100 percent.

Age-related eye disorders

Many changes to your vision that come with age you can adjust to. However, some changes may indicate the start of a serious eye disorder, which can lead to vision loss or permanent blindness if left untreated.

Blindness and low vision affects approximately one in 28 Americans older than age 40. The problems stem primarily from diseases such as macular degeneration, glaucoma and cataracts. Data from the 2000 U.S. census indicates that about 937,000 older adults experienced blindness and an additional 2.4 million had low vision. By the year 2020, blindness is expected to affect approximately 1.6 million Americans.

It may seem like there's little you can do to avoid certain eye disorders, but some may be prevented. Even disorders linked to factors such as heredity can often be slowed through early detection and treatment. That's why regular eye examinations are so important. Age-related eye disorders include:

Presbyopia. With the most common age-related vision problem, your lens gradually loses its elasticity and ability to change shape. As a result, it becomes more difficult to focus on objects without the help of corrective lenses (see page 163).

Macular degeneration. Over time, the macula — the part of the retina responsible for central vision — can deteriorate. Macular degeneration is the leading cause of blindness in Americans older than age 65. More than 7 million Americans are believed to be in early stages of the disease, and 1.75 million individuals are estimated to be in advanced stages. This figure is expected to increase to almost 3 million by 2020. Macular degeneration is most prevalent among whites of European descent.

Evidence suggests that you can take measures to delay the development of macular degeneration. A combination of antioxidant vitamins has been shown to reduce the risk of macular degeneration in an intermediate stage from progressing to a more advanced stage. Medications injected directly into the eye are effective at preserving central vision in individuals with the wet form of macular degeneration. For more on macular degeneration, see Chapter 2.

Glaucoma. Glaucoma is associated with increased pressure inside the eye. Left undetected, the condition can rob you of your vision — starting with your peripheral vision and eventually leading to blindness. It's estimated that the open-angle form of glaucoma affects more than 2 million Americans. Due to the aging population in the United States, that figure is expected to increase to more than 3 million by 2020.

If the disease is diagnosed early, damage often can be prevented or slowed with the use of eyedrops, which help reduce pressure within the eye. Laser treatment and surgery are options for more advanced stages of the disease. For more on glaucoma, see Chapter 4.

Cataracts. A cataract develops from the clouding of your normally clear lens. It's the leading cause of low vision in the United States. With age, almost everyone experiences cataracts to some degree. An estimated 20.5 million Americans older than age 40 have a cataract in either eye — a figure that's expected to rise to over 30 million by 2020. Surgery to remove the cataract and replace it with an artificial lens improves vision. For more on cataracts, see Chapter 5.

Eyelid problems. Changes in the eyelid tissues or muscles may cause eyelid problems. Sometimes, a condition progresses to the point where it begins to irritate the eye or impair vision. Surgery may be necessary to correct the problem. For more on eyelid conditions, see pages 148-154.

Dry eyes. Tears are essential lubricants for your eyes. Unfortunately, tear production and tear quality decrease with age, causing stinging, burning and scratchiness in the eyes. You can take a number of steps to minimize these symptoms. For more on dry eyes, see pages 155-158.

The eye exam

An eye examination involves a wide range of tests from simple tasks, such as reading a line of letters on a wall chart, to more complex tests, such as an automated machine that maps your loss of peripheral vision. You may not understand some of the technology being used during the examination. You may be asked to look through an endless array of lenses, and your eyes may be dilated and sensitive to light for several hours after the exam. Rest assured that each test is necessary.

The variety of tests allows your eye doctor to check different aspects of your vision, including visual acuity, peripheral vision, depth perception, color vision and the ability to focus on close objects. The tests also allow your doctor to detect a developing eye disorder and to assess whether any permanent damage has occurred. The following pages illustrate some of the more common tests involved in a typical eye exams. For more on eye exams, see pages 122-125.

The eye exam
External eye exam

An eye exam may start with a few simple questions about noticeable changes in your vision that are affecting your quality of life, as well as any eye problems you may be experiencing. Your doctor may begin by making a quick check of your eyes without use of any special instruments other than a light. He or she is checking:

- Your pupils to see if they respond normally
- The position and movement of your eyes, eyelids and lashes
- Your cornea and iris for clarity and shininess

The doctor may also assess the muscles that control eye movement, looking for weakness or poor control. He or she will study your eyes as you move them in specific directions and as you visually track a moving object, such as a pen being moved from side to side.

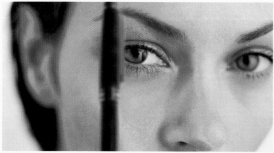

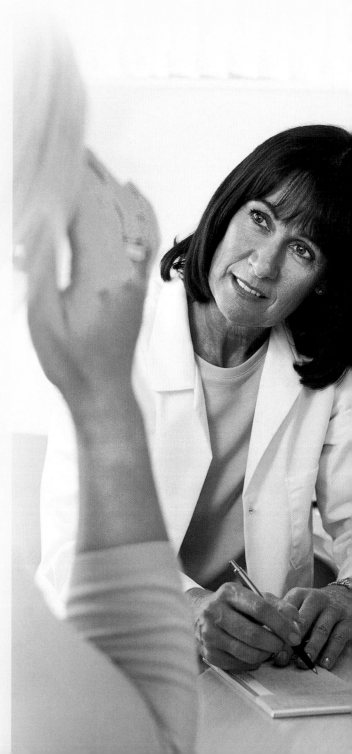

Visual field test (perimetry)

Your visual field includes everything that you can see without moving your eyes up, down, left or right. Perimetry shows whether you have difficulty with your peripheral vision — areas at the sides of your visual field. There are several types of visual field tests.

Confrontation exam. With one eye covered, you look at the doctor seated in front of you while he or she moves a hand in and out of your visual field. You indicate when you first see the hand.

Amsler grid. You focus on a black dot in the center of a black-line grid and describe whether any of the grid lines appear blurred, wavy or distorted (see also page 29).

Tangent screen exam. You sit at a short distance from a screen and stare straight ahead at the center of a target on the screen. You signal the technician whenever you see an object move into your peripheral vision.

Automated perimetry. You look at a testing screen on which small flashes of light blink on and off at different locations. Your job is to press a button each time you see a flash.

Test results map your responses and pinpoint gaps or blanks in your peripheral vision. These gaps may indicate eye disorders such as glaucoma, which has characteristic patterns of visual field loss (see also pages 95-96).

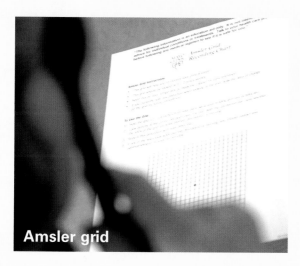

Amsler grid

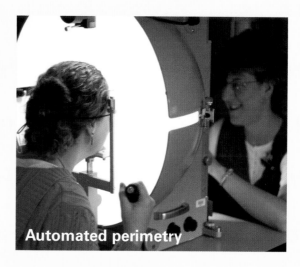

Automated perimetry

The eye exam
Visual acuity

Acuity refers to the sharpness of your vision or how well your eyes focus on an object. Your eye doctor may test your acuity by checking how well you can read the letters of the alphabet on a standard Snellen chart, positioned about 20 feet away. As you move down the chart, the lines of letters get smaller. Each eye is tested separately while the other one is covered.

Your eye doctor may also test how well you can read letters close up by having you read the smallest letter you can see on a card that's held 14 to 16 inches away from your eyes.

With the cover test, you're asked to look at an object in the room with one eye while the other eye is covered. The doctor observes the movement of the open eye and the amount of time required to focus on the object.

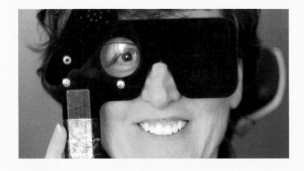

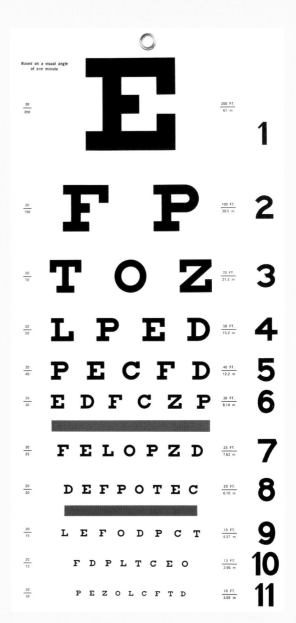

A Snellen chart is used to determine how well you can read letters from across the room. It's a common test for visual acuity.

Refraction assessment

Refraction refers to how light waves bend as they pass through your cornea and lens. The curvatures of the cornea and lens have to be just right for light to focus directly on your retina. If the curvature of either is too steep or too flat, the sharpest focus may occur before the light reaches your retina (nearsightedness) or at a point behind your retina (farsightedness). This assessment helps your eye doctor determine a corrective lens prescription to resolve a refractive error. If you don't need corrective lenses, you may not have a refraction assessment.

A computerized refractor is often used to measure the curvature of your eyes and estimate the prescription you need. Or your doctor may use a procedure called retinoscopy, in which he or she shines a light into your eye and approximates the prescription based on the light reflected by your retina.

Your doctor will likely fine-tune this assessment with a phoropter, a mask-like device that contains wheels of different lenses (shown below). You look at the Snellen chart through the phoropter and read aloud the smallest line of letters that you can see. After repeating this action several times with adjustments and different combinations, your doctor finds the lenses that give you the sharpest vision.

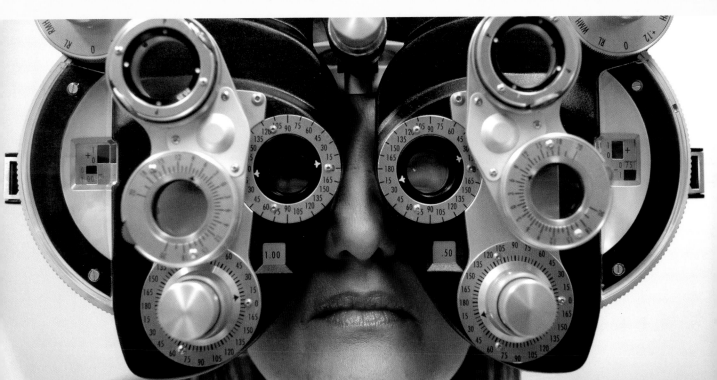

Slit lamp examination

A slit lamp allows a doctor to examine the structures at the front of your eye under high magnification. This specialized device is called a slit lamp because it uses an intense line of light — a slit — to provide oblique illumination of the cornea, iris, lens and anterior chamber. The instrument allows the doctor to view these structures in cross section and detect any small abnormalities.

Before the test, eyedrops are used to widen (dilate) your pupils and to numb the surface of the eye. In some cases, a camera may be attached to the slit lamp to take photographs of different parts of your eye.

For the test, your head is supported by forehead and chin rests positioned at the front of the slit lamp. When looking for corneal problems, your doctor also may use fluorescein dye. This dye spreads across your eye and glows bright yellow when hit with a blue light (light screened through a blue filter). This illumination highlights tiny cuts, scrapes, tears, foreign material or infections on your cornea.

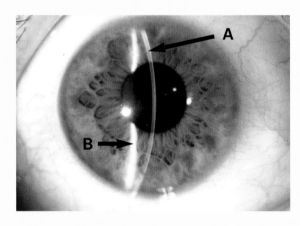

Slit-lamp examination
A slit of light is focused to provide an oblique view of the cornea (arrow A). The crescent of unfocused light on the left indicates the surface of the iris (arrow B). The doctor can also focus this light for a detailed view of the lens.

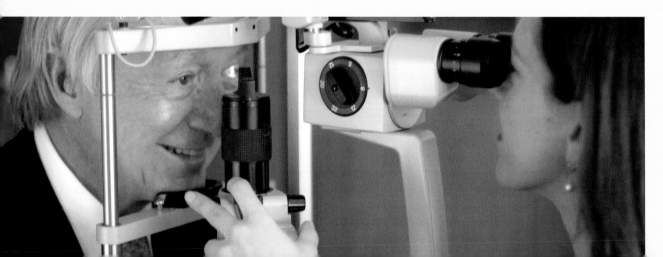

Retinal examination (ophthalmoscopy)

Ophthalmoscopy is an examination of the back of your eye, including your retina, optic disk and choroid. Your pupils are dilated beforehand with specialized eyedrops. Your doctor may use one or more techniques for this exam.

Direct examination. Your doctor shines a beam of light through your pupil and uses an ophthalmoscope to see the back of your eye. Sometimes, eyedrops aren't necessary to dilate your eyes before this exam.

Indirect examination. You may lie down or recline in a chair. The doctor holds the eye open and examines it with a bright light mounted on his or her forehead — a bit like a miner's lamp (photo on right). This exam lets your doctor see your eye in much greater detail and in three dimensions. Because of the bright light that's used, you're likely to see afterimages, but they disappear quickly.

Slit-lamp exam. The doctor looks through a small lens positioned in front of the eye along with a slit lamp to examine the retina, providing a very detailed view.

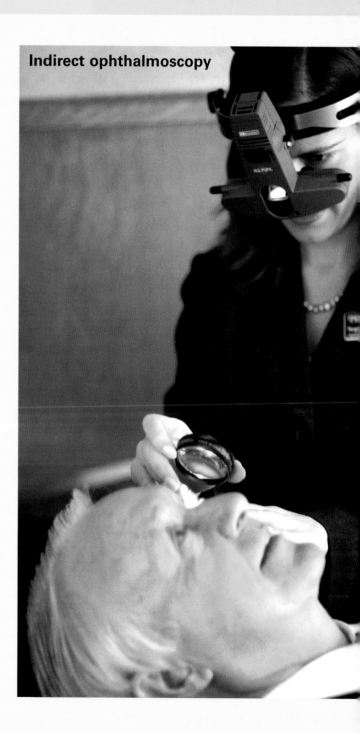

Indirect ophthalmoscopy

The eye exam
Glaucoma test (tonometry)

Tonometry measures your intraocular pressure — the pressure inside your eyes. This test helps your doctor detect the presence of glaucoma, a disease that causes intraocular pressure to build and can eventually result in blindness. Glaucoma can be treated if it's caught early. Various methods may be used to measure intraocular pressure.

Applanation tonometry. This test (shown below) measures the amount of force needed to temporarily flatten (applanate) a portion of your cornea. You receive eyedrops containing an anesthetic and fluorescein, an orange dye that makes the cornea easier to see under a blue light. Using a slit lamp equipped with the forehead and chin support apparatus, a tiny, flat-tipped cone gently touches your cornea. The procedure doesn't hurt, and the anesthetic wears off within about 20 minutes.

Noncontact tonometry. A machine uses a puff of air instead of the flat-tipped cone to test the pressure in your eye and calculate the intraocular pressure. No instruments will touch your eye, so you won't need an anesthetic. You'll feel mild pressure on your eye, which may feel a little uncomfortable but it lasts only seconds.

Pachymetry. This test measures the thickness of your cornea — an important factor in assessing intraocular pressure. After applying numbing eyedrops, your doctor uses an instrument that emits ultrasound waves to measure your corneal thickness.

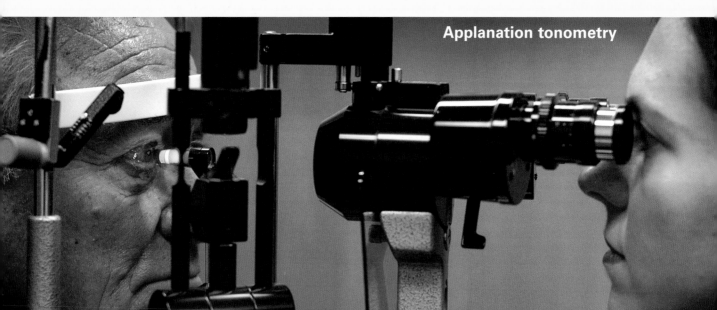

Applanation tonometry

Chapter 2

Macular degeneration

Age-related macular degeneration (AMD) is a chronic eye disease that develops when tissue in the macula begins to deteriorate. The result is blurred vision or a blind spot in your visual field. AMD tends to develop as you get older, hence the "age-related" part of its name.

In developed countries, macular degeneration is a leading cause of severe vision loss in people age 60 and older. An estimated 1.75 million Americans are in advanced stages of the disease. That number could increase to almost 3 million by 2020.

Macular degeneration affects your central vision but not your peripheral (side) vision; thus it doesn't cause total blindness. Still, the loss of clear central vision — critical for routine tasks such as reading, driving, preparing food and doing any type of detail work — greatly affects your independence and quality of life. The vision loss also may restrict your ability to interact and socialize with other people.

Although research hasn't provided a cure for macular degeneration, the future holds great promise. Several treatments exist that can effectively slow the most serious, vision-threatening stages of the disease. In recent years, a class of drugs has been developed that's capable not only of stopping macular degeneration but also of repairing damage to the macula that was once considered irreversible. This potential to reverse at least some of the vision loss offers hope for many individuals learning to live with the disease. Treatments for macular degeneration are discussed in later sections of the chapter.

Close-up look at the retina

The retina is a thin layer of tissue lining the inside back wall of the eyeball. It's packed with millions of light-sensitive cells and nerve cells that capture the light being focused on them by the cornea and lens, located at the front of the eye. The light-sensitive cells convert the light into impulses, which are sent to the brain via the optic nerve and interpreted as visual images.

Light-sensitive cells in the retina are either rod cells or cone cells. Rod cells are important for peripheral vision and help you see in dim light. Cone cells allow you to see sharp detail and distinguish colors but require good lighting in order to function well. Light striking the rods and cones triggers a chemical reaction, which generates electrical impulses that pass through the optic nerve.

At the center of the retina is the macula, which is the "high resolution zone" of your eye. Consisting primarily of cone cells, the macula is essential for clear visual acuity and allows you to see vivid colors and details. The small depression within the macula is called the fovea. The fovea consists of densely packed cone cells, and it provides your sharpest vision.

A layer of blood vessels underlying the retina is known as the choroid. These blood vessels supply oxygen and nutrients to the retina. The outermost surface of the retina, adjoining the choroid, is a layer of tissue called the retinal pigment epithelium (RPE). The RPE helps maintain the structural integrity of the retina and provides a passageway for nutrients moving from the choroid to the retina and for waste products moving from the retina to the choroid.

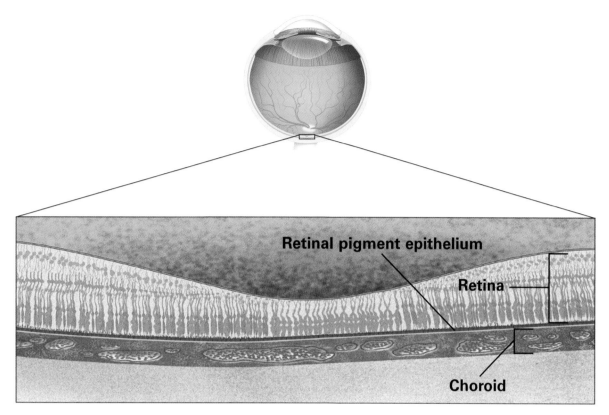

Cross section of the retina

The retinal pigment epithelium is a thin layer of tissue sandwiched between the photosensitive cells of the retina and the layer of blood vessels known as the choroid. The inset below is a cross-sectional photo of the retina and its underlying layers using a technique called optical coherence tomography. The fovea is the prominent indent on the surface of the retina. The choroid is the bright red layer beneath the retina.

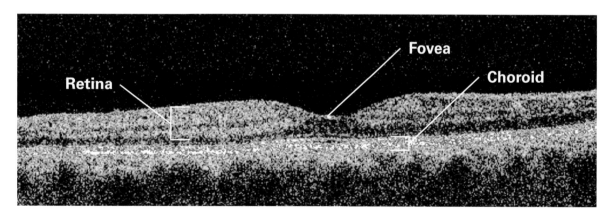

Signs and symptoms

Development of macular degeneration is generally a gradual and painless process, although the condition may sometimes progress rapidly. It can lead to severe loss of central vision in one or both eyes if left untreated. Depending on the type of macular degeneration you have — the dry form or the wet form — signs and symptoms may vary:

- Often one of the earliest signs of AMD is an increasing need for more light when reading or doing close-up work.
- Increasing difficulty adjusting to low illumination, such as when entering a dimly lit restaurant from the bright outdoors.
- Printed words, especially small type, become increasingly blurry.
- A decrease in the intensity and brightness of colors.
- Difficulty recognizing faces.
- Gradual haziness of your overall vision.
- Dark or blurry spots in your visual field (scotoma).
- An overall decline in your visual acuity.

- Need to scan your eyes all around to get an intact, complete outline of an object.
- Visual distortions (metamorphopsia), such as doorways or street signs that seem wavy or out of whack, and objects appearing smaller or farther away than they should be.

With macular degeneration, your vision may falter in one eye while the other remains fine for years. You may not notice any change because your good eye does such a good job of compensating for the weak one. Your vision — and your lifestyle — may be dramatically affected once this condition develops in both eyes.

Some people with severe vision loss may start to experience visual hallucinations, such as unusual patterns, geometric figures, animals or even grotesque-appearing faces. While the hallucinations may be frightening, they're not a sign of mental illness. In fact, these hallucinations are so common that there's a name for this phenomenon — Charles Bonnet syndrome. Should you experience these symptoms, you're encouraged to discuss them with your doctor or friends and family.

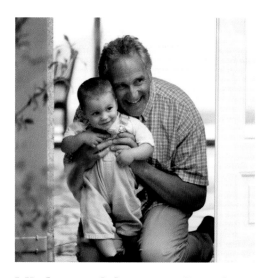 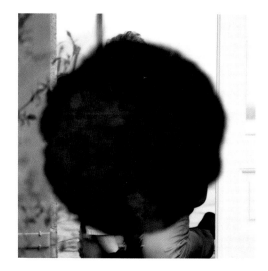

Vision with macular degeneration

In day-to-day activities with family and friends (normal vision shown at left), your eyesight will be impaired by a general haziness as macular degeneration develops. A blind spot typically forms at the center of your visual field (shown at right).

Causes

Macular degeneration often occurs following a deterioration of the thin, underlying layer of tissue known as the retinal pigment epithelium (RPE). The RPE weakens with age, and a weakened RPE is associated with breakdowns of vital nutritional and waste-removing cycles taking place between the retina and the choroid. Although the reasons why these systems stop functioning are poorly understood, the breakdowns may be triggered by a combination of factors.

As healthy, functioning tissue, the light-sensitive rods and cones in the macula continuously shed used-up outer segments as waste. This waste is processed in the RPE and moved into the choroid for disposal. At the same time, the rods and cones continue to produce new outer segments to replace the discarded ones.

Aging slows the waste-removal system to a point where the discarded outer segments start to accumulate in the RPE. This accumulation interferes with normal function of the light-sensitive cells in the macula, causing them to degenerate. Damaged cells can no longer send normal signals through the optic nerve to your brain, and your vision becomes blurred.

A sign that the waste-removal system is breaking down is the appearance on the retina of mottled pigmentation and drusen — clumps of waste deposit. The normal orange-red coloration of the retina assumes an uneven, splotchy appearance as areas of the RPE waste away — often in sharply defined circular shapes (geographic atrophy) — exposing the underlying choroid. The appearance of small drusen is common as you age, but the drusen generally don't interfere with vision. Large drusen with indistinct edges are of greater concern. They may merge together, involve the macula and affect your central vision.

A critical development in macular degeneration is the growth of abnormal blood vessels from the choroid, a process known as choroidal neovascularization (CNV). Unlike normal blood vessels, the abnormal ones are fragile and easily torn, leaking blood. The accumulating fluid lifts up sections of the retinal pigment epitheli-

um. For a visual analogy, think of tree roots growing under a sidewalk and lifting it up, creating an uneven, irregular surface to walk on. The swellings and blisters that form in the RPE damage the light-sensitive cells of the overlying macula.

Why CNV occurs isn't fully understood, but the presence of abnormal blood vessels further complicates other processes that damage the RPE, such as the breakdown of the waste-disposal system. Eventually, the abnormal vessels may transform into scar tissue, creating permanent blind spots in your visual field.

Scientists have identified several types of molecules (angiogenic factors) circulating in the bloodstream that cause new blood vessels to grow. One example is a protein called vascular endothelial growth factor, or VEGF. There are other molecules in the bloodstream that prevent blood vessels from growing called anti-angiogenic factors. Normally, the body maintains a delicate balance between the two types of molecules. Choroidal neovascularization occurs when this balance is disrupted, and angiogenic factors exceed anti-angiogenic factors.

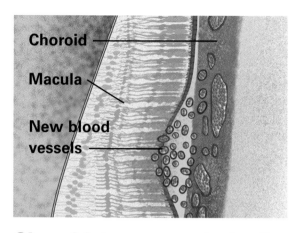

Choroidal neovascularization

As abnormal new blood vessels grow underneath the retinal pigment epithelium, some blood vessels eventually work their way through the thin layer of tissue and into the macula, where leaked fluid accumulates and destroys the photosensitive cells.

Risk factors

While researchers don't know the exact causes of age-related macular degeneration, they have identified a number of factors that appear to increase your risk of the disease. These factors include:

- **Age.** In the United States, AMD is the leading cause of severe vision loss in individuals age 60 and older.
- **Family history.** If someone in your family has, or had, macular degeneration, you have a higher risk of AMD. In recent years, researchers have identified several genes that may account for this inheritance.
- **Race.** AMD is more common in whites than in other ethnic groups, especially after age 75.
- **Sex.** Women are more likely than men are to develop AMD, and because they tend to live longer, women are more likely to experience severe vision loss from having the disease.
- **Cigarette smoking.** Exposure to cigarette smoke doubles your risk of macular degeneration. Smoking is the single most preventable cause of the disease.
- **Obesity.** Being severely overweight increases the chance that early or intermediate AMD will progress to a more advanced form of the disease.
- **Light-colored eyes.** People with light-colored eyes appear to be at greater risk than are those with darker colored eyes.
- **Exposure to sunlight.** It's possible that long-term exposure to sunlight may increase your risk of developing macular degeneration, but this risk has not been proved and remains controversial.

- **Low levels of certain nutrients.** This includes low blood levels of minerals such as zinc, and vitamins such as A, C and E.
- **Cardiovascular disease.** Conditions such as high blood pressure, stroke, heart attack and coronary artery disease can affect the blood supply to the eyeball.

Screening and diagnosis

Regular screenings may detect early signs of macular degeneration before the disease leads to vision loss. You should consult your eye doctor if you notice any changes to your central vision or your ability to distinguish colors and fine detail, particularly if you're older than age 50. Macular degeneration, particularly in its advanced stages, may progress rapidly, and the sooner you receive treatment, the better your chances of limiting vision loss.

To determine whether you have macular degeneration, you'll need to undergo a complete eye examination. Part of the examination will include testing with an Amsler grid. If you have macular degeneration, when you look at the straight lines of the grid some of the lines will seem faded, broken or distorted.

The examination will also include a close look at the back of your eye, after it has been dilated, with either a slit lamp or ophthalmoscope (see pages 18-19). Your doctor checks for mottled pigmentation and the presence of waste deposits (drusen) on the retina — and in particular, on the macula. He or she will also look for leaking (hemorrhaging) of blood or fluid in the macula.

Other diagnostic tests include fluorescein angiography to detect changes in pigmentation or the existence of abnormal blood vessels in your macula, which may not be visible with a slit-lamp exam (see page 47). A similar procedure called indocyanine green angiography may confirm or provide additional information to the fluorescein angiogram. Optical coherence tomography, also known as an OCT, creates a cross-sectional image of the eyeball to reveal areas where the retina has thickened or thinned, as well as if fluid has accumulated under the retina (see page 49).

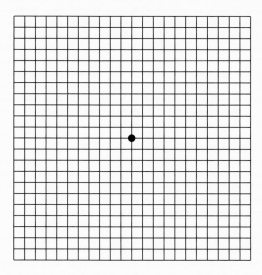 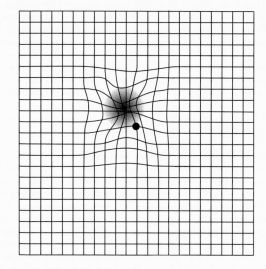

Visual symptoms of macular degeneration

Viewing an Amsler grid in the advanced stages of macular degeneration (right), you may see distorted grid lines or a blank spot near the center of the grid.

Amsler grid

You can monitor your vision with regular home checkups using an Amsler grid. This simple test can help you detect changes in your eyesight that you otherwise may not notice. To remind you to do the test, hang the grid someplace where you'll see it often — for example, on your refrigerator or alongside the bathroom mirror.

Here's how you perform the test:
- Hold the grid about 14 inches in front of you in good light. Use corrective lenses or reading glasses if you normally wear them.
- Cover one eye.
- Look directly at the center dot on the grid with your uncovered eye.
- While remaining focused on the dot, note whether all of the lines of the grid appear to be straight, complete (unbroken) and of similar contrast.
- Repeat the above steps using your other eye.
- If any part of the grid is missing or looks wavy, blurred or dark, contact your doctor immediately.

Although genetic abnormalities have been identified in some people with macular degeneration, genetic screening tests currently aren't being used to diagnose the disorder. However, in the future, they may be used to assess early risk.

Dry vs. wet

There are two major types of macular degeneration, commonly known as "dry" and "wet."

Dry macular degeneration. Dry macular degeneration occurs when the retinal pigment epithelium (RPE) begins to shrink (atrophy), characterized by mottled pigmentation and drusen that resemble yellow dots on a color photograph of the retina. Most people with macular degeneration have the dry form. In fact, AMD always starts out as the dry form. Dry AMD may initially affect only one eye, but in most cases, both eyes become involved.

In spite of these developments, you may notice little or no change in your vision at first. Many people who've received a diagnosis of early-stage dry macular degeneration aren't bothered by symptoms such as blurred eyesight, unless they live to a very old age. But as the drusen and mottled pigmentation continue to develop, vision gradually deteriorates. The thinning of the RPE may progress to a point where this protective layer disappears altogether, and may result in a complete loss of central vision.

Based on this progression, the dry form of macular degeneration is categorized in three stages:

Early stage. Several small drusen or a few medium-sized drusen are detected on the macula in one or both eyes. Generally, there's no vision loss in the earliest stage.

Intermediate stage. Many medium-sized drusen or one or more large drusen are detected in one or both eyes. Some people may notice blurring of their central vision at this stage. More lighting may be necessary for reading or detail work.

Advanced stage. In addition to drusen, the advanced stage involves an extensive breakdown of light-sensitive cells in the macula, causing a distinct

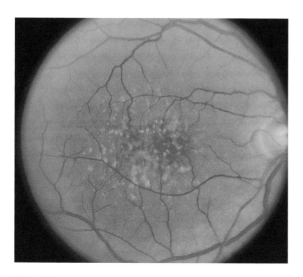

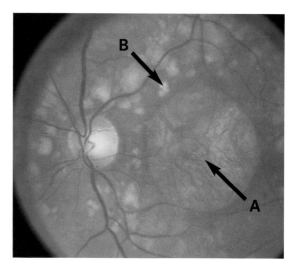

Early-stage dry macular degeneration

The hallmark of early-stage dry macular degeneration is the development of drusen on and around the macula. The drusen appear as yellow spots on color photographs of the retina.

Advanced-stage dry macular degeneration

The retinal pigment epithelium at the center of the retina has thinned and, in some areas, disappeared, exposing choroid blood vessels (arrow A). Large drusen, as indicated by arrow B, surround the macula.

blurry spot to appear in your central vision. This spot may increase in size and become denser or more opaque as the disease develops.

Although drusen aren't thought to cause vision loss, their size and number are key indicators of your risk of advanced disease, and even of developing the wet form of AMD.

Wet macular degeneration. The wet form of macular degeneration is

thought to account for only about 15 percent of all cases, but it's responsible for most of the severe vision loss experienced by people with AMD. If you develop wet macular degeneration in one eye, your odds of getting it in the other eye increase greatly.

Almost everyone with the wet form of the disease started out with the dry form. The dry form may turn into the wet form at any time, sometimes rather suddenly and at an early stage.

At the same time, it's possible for the dry form to develop into an advanced stage without ever becoming the wet form.

Wet macular degeneration develops as a result of choroidal neovascularization (CNV) — growth of abnormal blood vessels underneath the macula. The wet designation is due to fluid leaking from the fragile vessels, forming what looks like blisters or bumps under the macula. Eyes with the wet form of AMD also show signs of the dry form — that is, drusen and mottled pigmentation on the retina.

Ophthalmologists use fluorescein angiography to identify different patterns of CNV:

Occult. This term refers to the presence of abnormal blood vessels and the leakage of blood underneath the protective RPE layer. The condition progresses slowly and its presence may be disguised by other factors, making it difficult to locate the abnormal vessels. CNV may have a stippled appearance on a fluorescein angiogram.

Classic. The abnormal blood vessels have started to grow through the

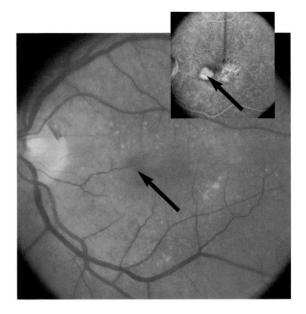

Wet macular degeneration

The arrow on the color photograph of the retina indicates where abnormal blood vessels have leaked fluid under the macula. A fluorescein angiogram of the same eye allows the doctor to accurately detect the full extent and the boundaries of the leaked fluid (arrow on inset).

RPE, increasing the amount of macular damage. The presence of classic CNV is obvious from the brightness of the fluorescein dye (hyperfluorescence) on the angiogram.

Mixed. Sometimes, a fluorescein angiogram reveals the presence of both occult and classic patterns of CNV in the retina. This condition

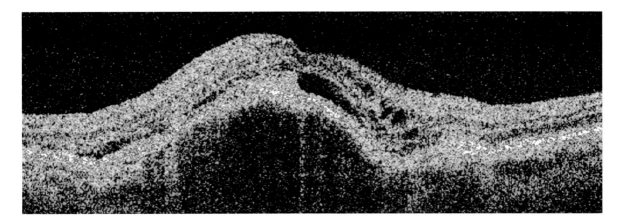

Retinal pigment epithelial detachment

An image of the retina taken with optical coherence tomography shows the elevation of the RPE by fluid accumulation in the choroid (the red layer).

may be identified as either "predominantly classic" or "minimally classic" forms.

A form of wet macular degeneration called retinal pigment epithelial detachment (PED) occurs when fluid leaking from the choroid elevates — or forms a bubble on — the RPE (see photo above). However, abnormal blood vessels may or may not have developed. When abnormal blood vessels are present, the condition is called fibrovascular PED. Your vision can remain relatively stable with PED for many months — or even years — before it slowly begins to deteriorate.

Treatment

In the past, treatment for macular degeneration focused primarily on preserving existing vision and preventing further loss, rather than on improving vision. Doctors made attempts to slow the disease, but damage to vision that may have already occurred was believed to be irreversible.

New research is gradually changing how the disease is treated. Permanent vision loss is no longer considered an inevitable consequence of macular degeneration. New treatments, if administered early in the course of the disease, may repair some of the damage and improve vision. That's why the earlier the diagnosis, the better your chance that you'll retain some functional vision.

In the early to intermediate stage, most people with macular degeneration have the dry form of the disease. Although this form has proved to be the most difficult to treat, risk of severe vision loss isn't as high as with the wet form. Because the dry form often progresses slowly, many people with the condition are able to continue living relatively normal, productive lives, especially if only one eye is affected.

Although people in the advanced stages of dry macular degeneration, or

Choosing the best course of treatment

What therapy is used to treat wet macular degeneration is generally determined by what stage of the disease you have. A thorough examination of the retina and the eye's underlying structures can help your doctor determine the best treatment choice.

One factor that your doctor looks at is the pattern of choroidal neovascularization — whether the blood vessels are hidden in an occult form (under the RPE) or exposed in a classic form (above the RPE).

Another critical factor is the location of the choroidal neovascularization (CNV) — whether it is away from the fovea (extrafoveal), alongside the fovea (juxtafoveal) or directly under the fovea (subfoveal). Treatment of subfoveal CNV can be more complex because the fovea is so critical for central vision.

A third factor in determining treatment is identifying the boundaries of the CNV — whether they're well-defined or poorly defined. It's easier and safer to use a laser to treat extrafoveal CNV that's contained within clearly identified boundaries, than it is to attempt to seal off abnormal blood vessels across a wide, diffuse area.

with untreated wet macular degeneration, can experience severe vision loss, it doesn't mean total blindness. Although the loss of central vision places severe restrictions on a person's independence and functional abilities, individuals still retain the ability to see light and use peripheral vision.

Should macular degeneration be detected, retina specialists may use one treatment or a combination of treatments to get the best results. All risks, benefits and possible complications of these procedures should be discussed with your doctor.

Treating dry macular degeneration

There was no effective treatment for dry macular degeneration until the release of the Age-Related Eye Disease Study (AREDS), which provided a clear direction for slowing the disease's progress. The study found that a daily supplement containing high doses of vitamin C, vitamin E, beta carotene (often vitamin A), zinc and copper reduced the risk of macular degeneration advancing to a more severe stage by up to 25 percent. For more information on AREDS, see pages 135-137.

Research on other potential treatments is currently under way. A new study just getting started — AREDS2 — will examine the effects of the antioxidants lutein and zeaxanthin and omega-3 fatty acids in halting or slowing progression of macular degeneration (see page 138).

Treating wet macular degeneration

Anyone noticing dark spots or wavy visual distortions in his or her visual field may be experiencing the onset of wet macular degeneration. These symptoms are caused by blood and fluid that has leaked from blood vessels and pooled under the RPE, elevating small sections of tissue in bubbles or blisters. Left untreated, the abnormal blood vessels typically grow larger and continue to leak more blood and fluid, causing more severe vision loss.

Even if treatment can't cure or prevent the disease, it can often halt or slow the disease's progression, allowing you to retain a useful portion of your vision. Meanwhile, a number of experimental therapies that offer real hope for limiting the effects of AMD are on the horizon.

Laser therapy. Laser therapy, or macular photocoagulation, is used to seal leaking blood vessels and stop the growth of new ones. Only a small percentage of people with macular degeneration are actually eligible for this type of treatment. For one thing, laser surgery can only be used on individuals who have the wet form of macular degeneration — estimated to be about 15 percent of all people with AMD. In addition, the area where the choroidal neovascularization is located must be well-defined and not under the fovea (extrafoveal), which isn't the case with many individuals.

For this therapy, a surgeon uses a high-energy ("hot") laser beam to create small burns in areas containing

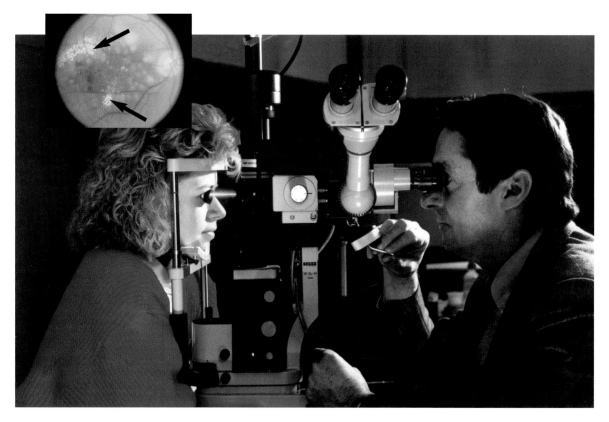

Laser photocoagulation

A special lens placed on the eye (left) focuses laser light to stop the growth of abnormal blood vessels under the retina and seal off the leakage of blood and fluid. Scar tissue forms at the location of each laser burn on the retina (see arrows on inset photo).

abnormal blood vessels. This seals off the vessels and prevents further damage. The entire process may take five to 10 minutes (see also pages 61-63).

The risk of the procedure is collateral damage from the laser, which destroys the photoreceptor cells of the macula that lie directly over the CNV. A scar forms at the location of each laser burn, and this scar can create a permanent blind spot in your vision.

Another downfall of the procedure is that CNV that's successfully destroyed has a tendency to recur. And often the recurrence is under the fovea (subfoveal). In this case, repeat laser treatment isn't an option because you don't want to destroy the fovea.

A decision to use laser therapy requires a careful consideration of the possible benefits vs. the potential risks. On one hand, if wet macular degeneration is left untreated, vision loss will likely continue to get more severe. On the other hand, laser therapy may slightly worsen vision or improve it only for a short time. The overall health of the macula and the presence of other health concerns also may play roles in determining whether to use laser therapy.

Photodynamic therapy. Photodynamic therapy (PDT) is used for treating abnormal blood vessels that are underneath the fovea (subfoveal) or next to the fovea (juxtafoveal). PDT combines a cold (nonthermal) laser and a light-sensitizing (photosensitizing) drug that's injected into your bloodstream. Verteporfin (Visudyne) is the only photosensitizing drug approved by the Food and Drug Administration for the treatment of choroidal neovascularization. When injected in the arm, verteporfin travels through the bloodstream and concentrates in the abnormal vessels of the retina. The dye doesn't stay in healthy tissue, which is unaffected by the laser.

When the surgeon directs cold-laser light at the treatment area, the photosensitizing drug is activated, causing a photochemical reaction that damages and closes off the abnormal blood vessels. Furthermore, damage to the overlying rod and cone cells of the macula is minimal and central vision is largely maintained. The CNV transforms into a thin scar. Photodynamic therapy can be repeated at three-month intervals if the abnormal vessels don't close or if the blood vessels later reopen.

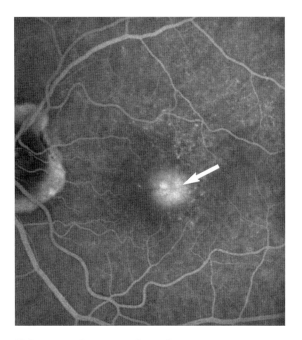 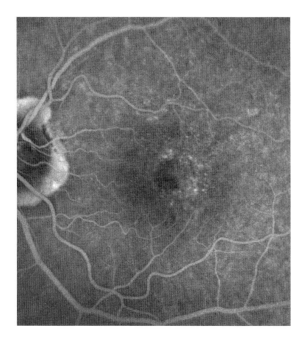

Photodynamic therapy

The image at right shows submacular leakage from abnormal blood vessels (see arrow). The image at left is the same eye following PDT showing a disappearance of the leakage.

Generally, PDT is most effective at the early stages of macular degeneration. Because the photosensitizing drug stays in your body for a while, you must stay out of the sun for several days following treatment or risk severe sunburn.

Anti-angiogenic therapies. At certain times, formation of new blood vessels in the body is normal. For example, following an injury, when damaged tissue is healing, new blood vessels will form. This process, known as

angiogenesis (an-jee-o-JEN-uh-sis), is triggered by the action of proteins, such as the vascular endothelial growth factor (VEGF), that signal blood vessel cells to grow.

A new approach to treating wet macular degeneration is to prevent the growth of abnormal blood vessels, rather than waiting to treat the problem once it has occurred. The drugs developed for this type of therapy are called anti-angiogenic medications. They work by inhibiting

Intravitreal injection

Anti-angiogenic drugs are delivered to the eye via injections directly into the vitreous. This is the most effective way to administer medications to the retina because they reach the target directly. When other means are used to administer the drug, for example, injection through the bloodstream, a much smaller amount reaches the retina and much larger doses are needed to be effective.

The risk of complications from intravitreal injection is low, and the problems are usually temporary and treatable. The most common side effect is redness and scratchiness of the eyeball. The most serious complication is endophthalmitis, a severe infection of the interior of the eyeball. Other possible complications include retinal detachment, intraocular hemorrhage and ocular hypertension. In rare instances, the drug triamcinolone acetonide may lead to development of a cataract.

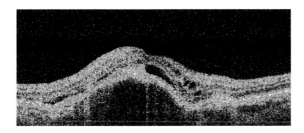 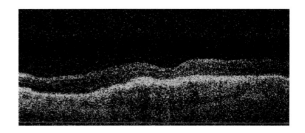

Anti-angiogenic therapy

The image at left, taken with optical coherence tomography, shows swelling and the accumulation of fluid in the macula. The image at right shows the same area of the retina after receiving anti-angiogenic treatment.

proteins that trigger the vascular growth process, such as VEGF. The treatment is ongoing — since the body continues to produce VEGF — and medications are administered at regular intervals.

This form of therapy resolves several problems associated with laser therapy. First, anti-angiogenic treatment can be used for a broader range of people, not just for individuals with CNV located outside the fovea.

Second, anti-angiogenic therapy is much less likely to cause vision loss. Laser therapies may close off abnormal blood vessels, but generally at the cost of additional damage to your vision. Each pulse of the laser destroys a small part of the retina overlying the CNV.

Drugs used in anti-angiogenic therapy include:

Pegaptanib. Pegaptanib (Macugen) was approved by the Food and Drug Administration in 2004 for treatment of wet macular degeneration. It targets a specific subtype of the vascular endothelial growth factor (VEGF-165) protein. By inhibiting VEGF-165, the drug can stop or slow vascular formation. Clinical trials demonstrated that vision loss was reduced by 70 percent in participants who used Macugen. It was effective with all forms of wet AMD.

Macugen is administered as a series of injections into the vitreous every six weeks and is generally well tolerated. Despite Macugen's positive results, Lucentis, another drug with better outcomes, is generally the first choice for anti-angiogenic therapy.

Ranibizumab. Ranibizumab (Lucentis) was approved by the Food and Drug Administration in July 2006 for treating wet macular degeneration. Like Macugen, this drug can halt the growth of abnormal blood vessels by inhibiting the activity of the VEGF protein. Unlike Macugen, Lucentis inhibits all subtypes of the protein, not just VEGF-165. Lucentis is injected into the vitreous once a month. In clinical trials, vision stabilized or improved in 95 percent of participants receiving the medication after 12 months of use.

The most common side effects from taking Lucentis may include conjunctival hemorrhage, eye pain, floaters, increased eye pressure and eye inflammation.

Bevacizumab. Some doctors are prescribing bevacizumab (Avastin), a drug closely related to Lucentis, which, so far, shows promising results. Avastin also is administered by injection into the eye. Using Avastin to treat AMD is considered an off-label use, as it's generally used for colon and rectal cancer. Currently, there's an ongoing trial comparing Avastin and Lucentis.

Drug therapies under study. Angiostatic therapy involves a different class of drugs that show promise in the treatment of macular degeneration. These drugs are forms of steroids that are capable of stopping the abnormal growth of new blood vessels in the retina — but in a slightly different manner than anti-angiogenic drugs.

Triamcinolone acetonide. The steroid medication triamcinolone acetonide (Kenalog) is used to treat eye inflammation and swelling (edema). Ongoing studies are analyzing if the drug might improve vision in people with macular degeneration. When used in combination with photodynamic therapy, triamcinolone helps reduce the number of times you need re-treatment. It also may help limit damage to the retina caused by photodynamic therapy.

Anecortave acetate. Study results show that the effectiveness of anecortave acetate (Retaane), another angiostatic drug, compares favorably to that of photodynamic therapy. Researchers are also evaluating whether Retaane can stop or slow the transition of dry macular degeneration to wet macular degeneration.

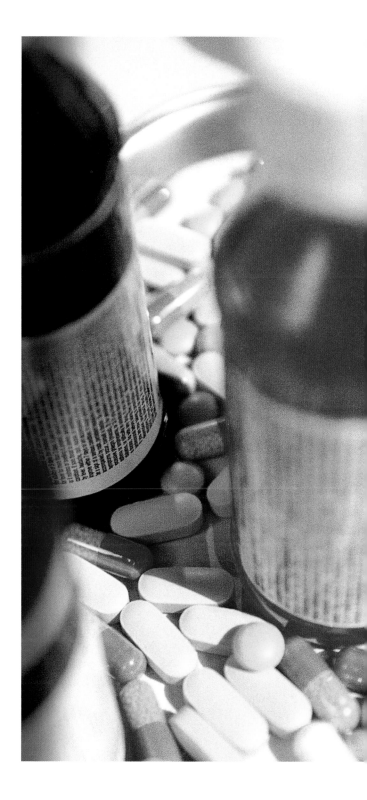

Also undergoing study is the angio-genetic inhibitor squalamine (Evizon), which is administered intravenously rather than injected directly into the vitreous. Other drugs under study include Sirna-027 and VEGF Trap.

Surgical treatments. Surgical treatments for macular degeneration are generally considered to be in their experimental stages. Definitive conclusions regarding their effectiveness await the results of further study.

With macular translocation surgery, the surgeon detaches the retina and relocates the fovea away from an underlying area of choroidal neovascularization (CNV) to an area of healthy tissue. Abnormal blood vessels growing within the fovea are removed with a small forceps or laser. Macular translocation may be performed if vision loss is recent, the extent of CNV is limited and the tissue around the fovea is healthy. If the overlying photoreceptor cells in the macula still function, it's possible to recover some vision after surgery.

Another experimental procedure is submacular surgery, which involves making a small incision in the retina and removing the underlying CNV with a small forceps. However, this procedure may only be used for CNV located between the macula and the retinal pigment epithelium — most CNV lies between the RPE and the choroid. Results of a recent submacular surgery study have cast further doubt on the use of this procedure for macular degeneration.

Prevention

There's nothing you can do to change your race or genetic makeup or keep you from getting older — all major risk factors for age-related macular degeneration. But the following measures may help prevent or delay development of the disease. The earlier you can start these measures, the better — before the condition develops and causes irreversible damage to your vision.

Eat foods containing antioxidants. A nutritionally balanced diet with plenty of fruits and vegetables, particularly leafy greens, may be among the most important factors in promoting good retinal health (see pages 134-140). The results of the Age-Related

Eye Disease Study (AREDS) suggest that you should include foods containing antioxidants in your diet. Antioxidants prevent oxidative damage to tissue such as the retina. Look for foods rich in vitamins A, C and E, including carrots, broccoli, spinach, tomatoes, sweet potatoes, citrus fruit, berries, cantaloupe, mango, whole-grain products, wheat germ and nuts.

Eat fish. Regular consumption of fish and the omega-3 fatty acids found in fish can result in a reduced risk of macular degeneration. Use discretion if you're considering more frequent consumption of fish; certain types may contain high levels of toxins and other contaminants.

Take supplemental vitamins and minerals. You may need to take supplements to reach the adequate levels of vitamins and minerals for your diet. These supplements can be purchased individually or in combination. But talk to your doctor before using any supplements, particularly in large doses. Unless your doctor instructs you otherwise, don't exceed the Recommended Dietary Allowance (RDA) for any substance.

Large doses may interact with other medications that you're taking, or they may not be right for you. For example, if you currently smoke or you're a former smoker, high doses of beta carotene (vitamin A) may

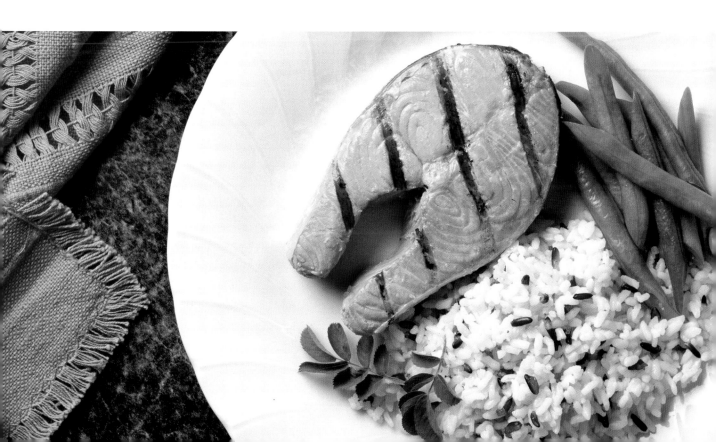

significantly increase your risk of lung cancer. If you also take a daily multivitamin, check the label to make sure that you don't exceed the RDAs for zinc and vitamins A, C and E.

Wear sunglasses that block out harmful ultraviolet light. Most ultraviolet (UV) light is filtered by the cornea and lens at the front of your eye. Still, it's safer to wear orange-, yellow- or amber-tinted sunglasses when you're outdoors. Look for glasses that filter 99 percent to 100 percent of ultraviolet A (UVA) and ultraviolet B (UVB) rays (see also pages 128-129).

Stop smoking. Smokers are more likely to develop macular degeneration than are nonsmokers. Ask your doctor for help to stop smoking.

Manage other diseases. For example, if you have cardiovascular disease or high blood pressure, take your medication and follow your doctor's instructions for controlling the condition.

Get regular eye exams. Early detection of macular degeneration increases your chances of preventing serious vision loss. If you're older than age 40, get an exam every two to four years, and if you're older than age 65, schedule an exam every year or two. If you have a family history of macular degeneration, have your eyes examined more frequently, perhaps annually.

Screen your vision regularly. If you've received a diagnosis of early-stage macular degeneration, your doctor may suggest that you regularly monitor your vision at home with an Amsler grid. Doing so may help you detect subtle changes in your vision at the earliest possible time and seek help promptly.

If you experience vision loss due to macular degeneration, your doctor can prescribe optical devices called low-vision aids that will help you see details better. Or your doctor may refer you to a low-vision specialist. In addition, a wide variety of support services and rehabilitation programs are available that may help you adjust your lifestyle.

Imaging the eye

If there's ever a concern at your next eye exam, the doctor may arrange for an imaging test of your eyes. Imaging tests are essential tools for detecting and diagnosing eye disease and for tracking the effectiveness of treatment. These sophisticated technologies provide precise, detailed pictures of structures or developments inside of your eye that might otherwise be hidden or difficult to see without surgery. Special filters or dyes are sometimes used with these tests to highlight specific types of information.

The following pages explain several imaging tests that are commonly used during eye exams, such as fundus photography, fluorescein angiography, ultrasonography and optical coherence tomography. The images from these tests often guide treatment decisions for many of the conditions described in this book. As the technologies continue to advance, doctors are getting more and higher quality information. And with the greater use of imaging technology, there's less need for exploratory surgery to detect disease.

In medical terminology, *fundus* describes the bottom or base inside a hollow organ. The fundus of the eye includes the retina and underlying layers, such as the choroid, located at the back of the eyeball. Fundus photographs are routinely taken to diagnose a wide variety of eye disorders and provide a valuable record of changes in the appearance of the retina.

For the test, you sit with your head supported by chin and forehead rests in front of the fundus device, which is a combination microscope and camera. The photographs are taken directly through the pupil opening. Specialized dyes and colored filters may be used for better contrast.

A healthy retina has an even, reddish hue. The optic disk is the yellowish-orange circular structure with blood vessels radiating from it (arrow A). The macula is the deep red spot at the center of the retina (arrow B). The lower image shows the development of a macular hole at the retina's center (arrow C) — see page 72.

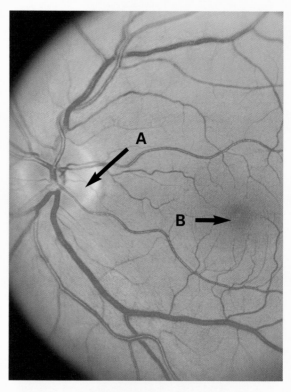

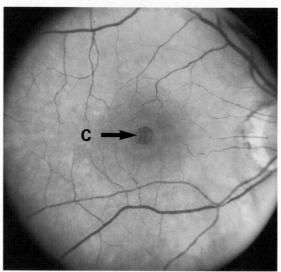

Fluorescein angiography

Fluorescein angiography is commonly used to study circulation patterns in the retinal blood vessels. The test uses the dye fluorescein (flooh-RES-ene) sodium and a special camera that filters out all visible wavelengths except for the dye color. The high-contrast, black-and-white images allow the doctor to see subtle or hidden features such as tissue swelling (edema) and tiny bulges on blood vessel walls (microaneurysms). The test also reveals new blood vessel growth (neovascularization) and the leakage of blood and fluid from tears in the vessel walls.

The testing procedure begins as fluorescein dye is injected into a vein of the arm. When the dye reaches the retinal blood vessels, the camera takes a rapid sequence of pictures that reveals how the dye circulates through the retinal capillaries.

The doctor may choose a dye that glows under a different wavelength of light in cases where fluorescein dye proves inadequate. For example, indocyanine green angiography may provide more detail of the choroid layer with the use of infrared light.

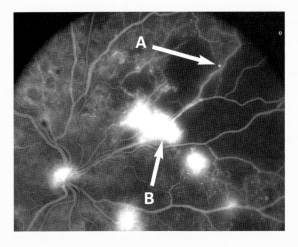

Tiny microaneurysms (white dots such as at arrow A) and subretinal hemorrhaging (clouded spots with indistinct edges such as at arrow B) show the development of diabetic retinopathy on this fluorescein angiogram.

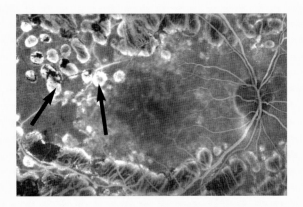

The arrows on this fluorescein angiogram indicate laser burns following treatment with photocoagulation on the retina.

Imaging the eye
Ultrasonography

Ultrasonography, or echography, uses sound waves to create an image of the eye's interior in the same way that sonar technology creates images of underwater objects. What's known as an A-scan is useful for measuring the size and shape of the eye. The B-scan provides a two-dimensional cross section of the eye and is useful for diagnosing retinal detachments, tumors and inflammation.

After administrating anesthetizing drops, a wand (transducer) is placed at the front of the eye that emits high-frequency sound waves. These waves bounce off internal structures and back to the transducer, which converts the reflected waves into an image — usually referred to as an ultrasound. The wavelengths vary according to the different densities of the tissue that the sound waves are striking.

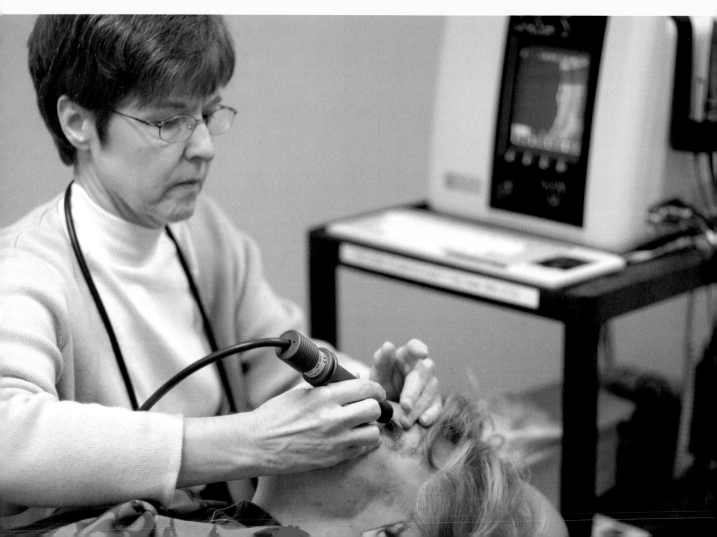

Optical coherence tomography

Optical coherence tomography (OCT) combines the principles of ultrasonography with the high-resolution performance of a microscope. OCT captures infrared lightwaves reflected off the internal structures of the eye, but with a resolution that's many times greater than what can be achieved with sound waves. The result is a detailed, cross-sectional image that clearly displays the well-defined boundaries of the retina and underlying layers.

False colors are added to the images to assist interpretation, with bright colors such as white, yellow and red corresponding to areas of high reflectivity and dark colors such as blue and black corresponding to areas of low reflectivity. The procedure is useful for checking the thickness (or thinness) of the retina and for diagnosing disorders such as macular holes, macular edema, macular degeneration and retinal inflammation.

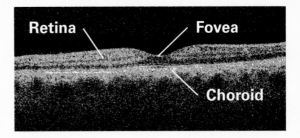

The OCT above is a cross section of a normal retina clearly showing the fovea and underlying choroid. The OCT below shows the result of choroidal neovascularization due to macular degeneration. Note the accumulation of subretinal fluid (arrow A), swelling and the formation of a large pigment epithelial detachment (arrow B).

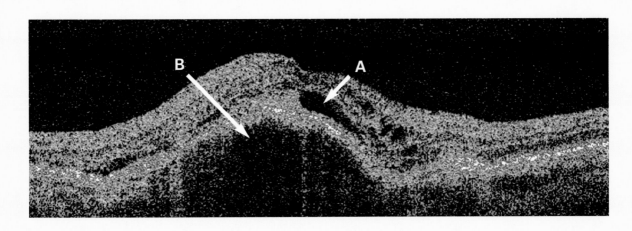

Detecting macular degeneration

A doctor diagnosing eye disease such as macular degeneration may employ several imaging technologies to get a comprehensive view of the retina. The color fundus photograph (left) shows a dark purplish patch under the macula, indicating where blood and fluid has leaked from abnormal blood vessels growing under the retina (arrow A). Small drusen are also present on the surface (arrow B). A fluorescein angiogram of the same retina (right) clearly shows the boundaries of the leaked fluid (arrow C).

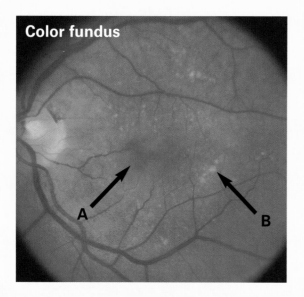

Color fundus

A

B

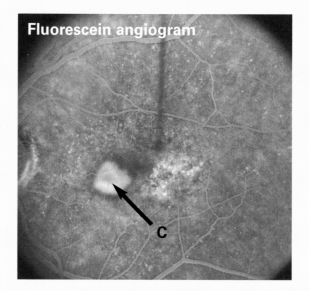

Fluorescein angiogram

C

Optical coherence tomography pro-vides a different view of the retina, revealing how the fluid has formed in cystoid pockets and caused swelling (arrow D). Smaller pockets of subretinal fluid are also forming (arrow E).

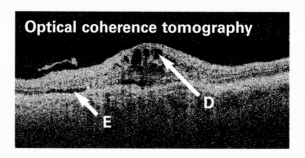

Optical coherence tomography

D

E

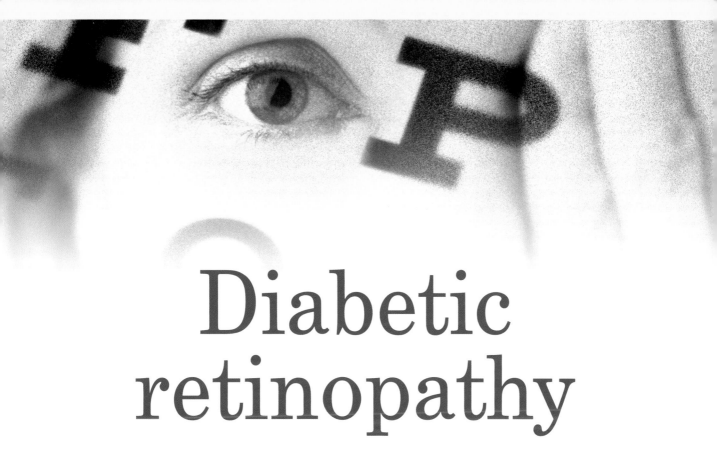

Chapter 3

Diabetic retinopathy

Vision loss is a major concern for people with diabetes. If not controlled, the condition can cause blindness. According to the American Diabetes Association, diabetes is the leading cause of new cases of blindness in adults ages 20 to 74.

The threat of blindness from diabetes may seem scary. But there's more

cause for hope than for alarm. With early detection and treatment, the risk of vision loss from diabetic retinopathy — the most serious eye complication of diabetes — is small. If you have diabetes, you can take steps to protect your sight. These include having a yearly eye examination and keeping your blood glucose and blood pressure under control.

Diabetes and your eyes

The term *diabetes* refers to a group of diseases that affect the way your body uses blood sugar — also called blood glucose — which is transported via your circulatory system. Glucose is vital to your health because it's the main source of energy for your body's cells. If you have diabetes, you have too much glucose in your blood, and excessive glucose can lead to serious problems.

There are two types of diabetes. With type 1 diabetes, your body produces little or no insulin, a hormone that's necessary for your cells to absorb and process glucose. With type 2 diabetes — the most common form of the disease — your body produces some insulin, but your cells are resistant to it. Most of the glucose stays outside the cells and accumulates in the bloodstream.

Diabetes is a systemic disorder, meaning that it affects your entire body, from head to toe. Long-term complications develop gradually and may lead to other disabling or life-threatening conditions, including cardiovascular disease, nerve damage, kidney failure, increased risk of infection and vision loss.

Retinopathy refers to a number of non-inflammatory conditions that affect the retina, including some that may lead to blindness. The root cause of retinopathy may be a disease such as diabetes or high blood pressure (hypertension). In the case of diabetes, too much glucose in the bloodstream damages blood vessels that supply nutrients to organs and tissues in the body, including the eyes. The tiny blood vessels (capillaries) located at the back of the eye are often among the first to be damaged.

Initially, the capillaries swell and leak fluid into the retina, causing your vision to blur. As the disease progresses, tiny new blood vessels grow out of the retina. These vessels may break and bleed into the clear vitreous that fills the interior of the eyeball, clouding your vision. Scar tissue also may form, causing the retina to detach from the back of the eye.

The longer you have diabetes, the more likely it is that you'll develop diabetic retinopathy. Nearly everyone with type 1 diabetes and more than six out of 10 people with type 2 diabetes who've had diabetes for 20 years develop some form of eye damage. Most people experience only mild vision problems. For others, the effects are more severe, including blindness.

Types of retinopathy

There are two types of diabetic retinopathy. Both types can be detected with an eye examination in which the doctor dilates the eye to closely study the retina. Usually both eyes are similarly affected, although the disease may become more advanced in one eye than in the other.

Nonproliferative type

Nonproliferative diabetic retinopathy (NPDR) is the most common form of the disease. It's also sometimes called background diabetic retinopathy. In NPDR, the walls of the retinal capillaries become weakened from high levels of glucose. Tiny bulges called microaneurysms (mi-kro-AN-u-rizmz) protrude from the vessel walls.

The microaneurysms may begin to leak, oozing blood into the retina.

Diabetic retinopathy may develop even if your diabetes is under control, but most often the symptoms tend to be mild and may not affect your ability to see. Vision problems from more severe NPDR are usually the result of swelling in the macula (macular

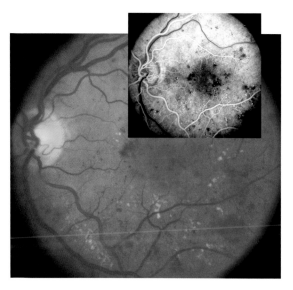

Nonproliferative diabetic retinopathy

Engorged blood vessels, microaneurysms (tiny red dots), hemorrhages (large red dots) and exudates (yellow spots) are commonly observed signs of NPDR. A fluorescein angiogram of the same eye (see inset) shows numerous microaneurysms as intense white dots. The dark spots are hemorrhages and exudates.

Signs of diabetic retinopathy

If diabetic retinopathy is present, a close examination of the retina generally reveals these characteristic signs:

Exudates. Fatty deposits resembling tiny cream-colored or yellow spots appear around the leaking walls of a retinal capillary. Exudates generally don't obscure vision unless they develop in the macula.

Cotton-wool spots. The tiny capillaries that nourish the retina are sometimes blocked off due to chronically high levels of blood glucose. Areas of the retina deprived of nourishment may suffer nerve damage, which appears as white, fluffy wisps on the surface. Tissue damage due to obstructed blood flow is referred to as ischemia.

Vitreous hemorrhage. Blood vessels growing in the retina (neovascularization) are fragile and easily ruptured, especially from the tugs and pulls of a shrinking vitreous. Blood from vessel ruptures and leaking microaneuryisms spills into the normally clear vitreous. Minor bleeding may produce a number of dark spots or floaters in your field of vision. More severe bleeding can cloud the vitreous, blocking the passage of light to the retina.

Bleeding into the vitreous, by itself, usually doesn't cause permanent vision loss. The blood eventually clears from the eye — usually within a few months — and your vision returns to its previous clarity, unless the retina has been damaged.

edema) or of the closing off of capillaries, reducing blood flow to the macula (macular ischemia). On photos, the macula is the reddish patch at the center of the retina (see page 7). When the macula can't function properly, your central vision blurs.

Proliferative type

Proliferative diabetic retinopathy (PDR) is a more advanced form of the disease. About half the people with very severe NPDR progress to PDR within one year.

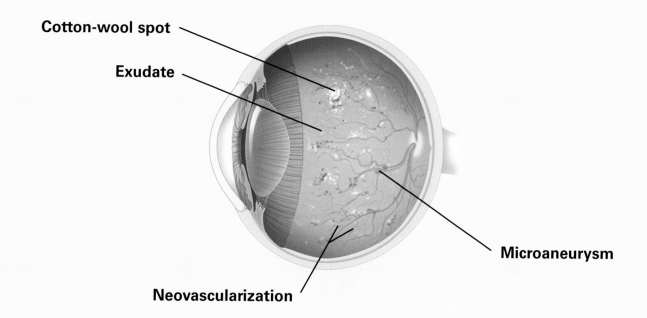

Cotton-wool spot

Exudate

Microaneurysm

Neovascularization

Macular edema. The most frequent cause of vision loss with nonproliferative diabetic retinopathy is from macular edema. Fluid from leaking capillaries accumulates in the macula, causing the tissue to swell. The fluid often forms in cyst-like pockets. Symptoms include blurred central vision and objects in your field of vision that appear to have wavy outlines.

Retinopathy becomes proliferative when abnormal new blood vessels grow, or "proliferate," on the retina or the optic nerve. These fragile blood vessels may also grow into the clear vitreous. The vessels begin to hemorrhage fluid and blood.

The abnormal growth of new blood vessels often follows a widespread closing off of capillaries in the retina due to high blood glucose levels. Unfortunately, these new blood vessels don't resupply oxygen-starved tissue with a normal blood flow.

Instead, they produce complications that affect both your central and peripheral vision. These may include:

Traction retinal detachment. New blood vessels in the retina are often accompanied by the growth of scar tissue on the retinal surface. This scar tissue shrinks and, as it shrinks, pulls the retina away from the underlying layers. In addition, as the vitreous shrinks due to aging, new blood vessels that have grown into and attached themselves to the vitreous tug on the retina. This tension, or "traction," may cause the retina to detach, forming blank or blurred areas in your visual field.

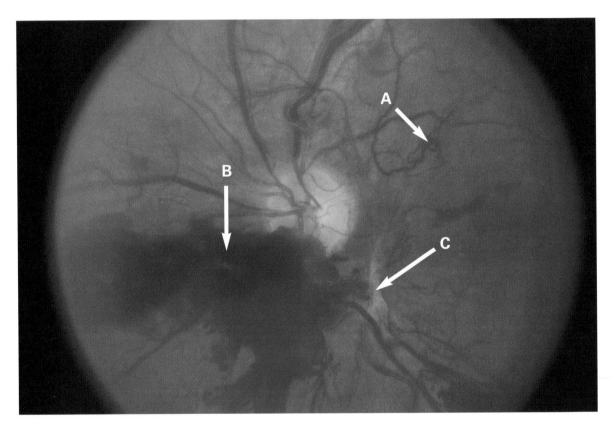

Late-stage proliferative diabetic retinopathy

In an advanced stage of PDR, abnormal blood vessels have grown on the optic nerve and retina and into the vitreous cavity (arrow A). These blood vessels break, causing massive hemorrhages (arrow B) and the formation of scar tissue (arrow C).

Neovascular glaucoma. Growth of new blood vessels in the retina may be accompanied by growth of new blood vessels on the iris. This increases intraocular pressure, causing a condition called neovascular glaucoma (for more on glaucoma, see pages 85-104). Because these changes at the front of the eye stem from problems at the back of the eye, this condition can be treated with procedures such as photocoagulation (see pages 36-37). If left untreated, neovascular glaucoma can cause pain, vision loss and, possibly, loss of the eye.

Signs and symptoms

In the early stages of diabetic retinopathy, most people will not experience any signs and symptoms. In fact, noticeable changes to your vision may not be evident until the disease has progressed to an advanced stage. The best way to detect diabetic retinopathy in its earliest and most treatable stage is to schedule regular eye exams.

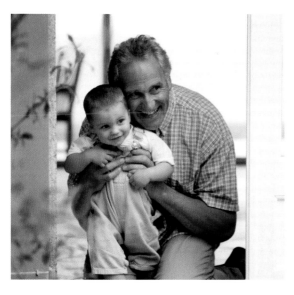 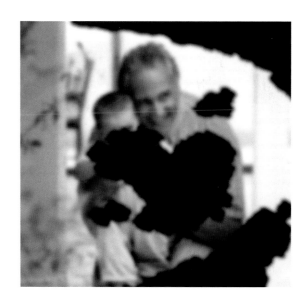

Vision with diabetic retinopathy

As diabetic retinopathy develops into more severe stages, your normal vision (shown at left) will become blurred and clouded from blood hemorrhaging into the vitreous (shown at right).

As the condition progresses to more advanced stages, visual symptoms may include:

- "Spiders," "cobwebs" or tiny specks floating in your visual field
- Dark streaks or a red film that blocks vision
- General vision loss, but in one eye more than the other
- Blurred vision that may fluctuate
- A dark or empty spot in the center of your visual field

- Poor night vision
- Difficulty adjusting from bright light to dim light

Risk factors

The National Eye Institute estimates that between 40 percent and 45 percent of Americans diagnosed with diabetes have some form of diabetic

Blurred vision with diabetes

Blurred vision is often caused by fluctuations in blood glucose levels. Prolonged periods of excessively high blood glucose can cause sugar and its breakdown products to accumulate in the lens of the eye. This accumulation makes the lens swell, resulting in nearsightedness — making distant objects appear blurry. The nearsightedness subsides once blood glucose is brought under control, and the lens can return to its normal size.

Blurred vision may also stem from macular edema or swelling, regardless of your blood glucose level. This is a cause for greater concern because untreated macular edema damages central vision. The swelling may fluctuate during the day, making your vision appear to get better or worse.

When new blood vessels form in the vitreous from proliferative diabetic retinopathy (PDR), the vessels may leak, causing dark spots to float in and out of your field of vision. Hazy clouds that blur your vision, caused by massive hemorrhaging into the vitreous, often follow the appearance of these floaters within a few days or weeks.

retinopathy. If you have diabetes, you're at risk of retinopathy, regardless of whether you have the type 1 or type 2 form. Your risk increases the longer you have the disease.

Generally, individuals with type 1 diabetes are at higher risk of retinopathy because they tend to become diabetic at a young age. If you were over age 30 when you developed diabetes, your risk is lower — although for some, retinopathy can be their first sign of diabetes. Regardless of your age, if you need to take insulin, your risk of retinopathy is increased.

Other risk factors include:
- Poorly controlled diabetes
- High blood pressure
- High blood cholesterol
- Obesity
- Kidney disease
- Pregnancy

Screening and diagnosis

A common misconception among people with diabetes is, "As long I can see well, there's nothing wrong with my eyes." That's false confidence. The signs and symptoms of diabetic retinopathy can be so subtle that many people are unaware of developing problems. Vision loss due to diabetic retinopathy often results from the fact that people didn't seek early medical attention. For this reason, regular eye examinations are very important.

The National Eye Institute recommends that if you have diabetes you receive a comprehensive dilated eye exam at least once a year. Dilation greatly enlarges your pupil, which gives the doctor a better view for studying your retina with a slit lamp or ophthalmoscope. People with diabetic retinopathy may need more frequent visits to the eye doctor.

In addition, if you have diabetes and become pregnant, you should have a comprehensive dilated eye exam as soon as possible. The doctor may recommend additional eye exams throughout your pregnancy.

See your eye doctor promptly if your vision becomes blurry, spotty or hazy. If diabetic retinopathy is found, the course of treatment will depend on the severity of the condition and whether your vision is currently impaired or threatened by the changes to the retina.

Your eye doctor will likely diagnose diabetic retinopathy — either nonproliferative or proliferative — if an eye examination reveals any of the following signs:

- Leaking blood vessels
- Retinal hemorrhage
- Swollen retina (edema)
- Fatty deposits (exudates) in the retina
- Nerve fiber damage (cotton-wool spots) in the retina
- Changes in blood vessels, such as closures, beading and loops
- Bulges in blood vessel walls (microaneurysms)
- Formation of new blood vessels (neovascularization)
- Vitreous hemorrhage
- Formation of scar tissue with retinal detachment

As part of the examination, your doctor may include tests such as fluorescein angiography and optical coherence tomography (see pages 47 and 49) to identify leaking blood vessels and swelling. These factors may be difficult to detect with the standard eye exam tests.

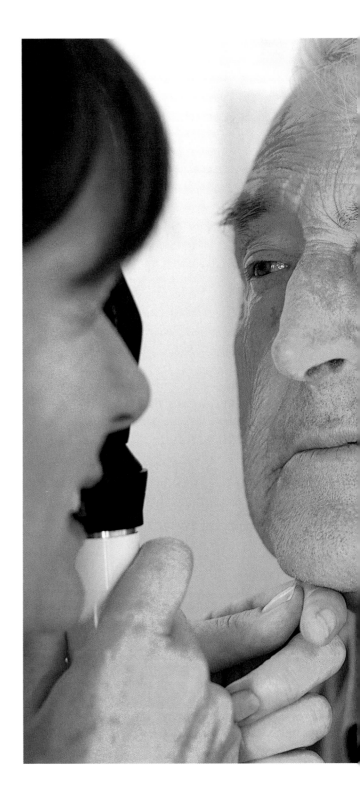

Treatment

If you are diagnosed with mild non-proliferative diabetic retinopathy, you may not require treatment immediately. However, your eye doctor will need to closely monitor any changes on your retina.

The more advanced stages of nonproliferative diabetic retinopathy as well as proliferative diabetic retinopathy require prompt treatment. The two main surgical procedures used to treat diabetic retinopathy are laser photocoagulation and vitrectomy. Most of the time, these treatments are effective and able to slow or stop progression of the disease for some time. But they're not a cure. Because diabetes is a systemic disorder and continues to affect your body, you may experience retinal damage and vision loss at a later time.

Anti-angiogenic drugs that inhibit or stop the growth of abnormal blood vessels provide a promising new therapy for diabetic retinopathy. Leakage from the abnormal blood vessels is a primary cause of macular swelling and vitreous hemorrhage, both of which lead to severe vision loss.

Laser photocoagulation

This procedure is used to stop the leakage of blood and fluid in the retina, thus slowing progression of the disease. The decision to use photocoagulation (fo-toe-ko-ag-u-LA-shun) will depend on the severity of your condition and how well your retina may respond to treatment.

Your doctor may recommend photocoagulation if you have:
- Swelling (edema) of the retina that involves the macula
- Severe stage of nonproliferative diabetic retinopathy, and you're unable to return for frequent follow-up visits
- Proliferative diabetic retinopathy
- Neovascular glaucoma

In photocoagulation, a high-energy laser beam burns small, pinpoint areas of the retina where leakage is taking place and seals off the abnormal blood vessels (see also pages 36-37). The procedure may take place in a doctor's office or an outpatient surgical center.

Before the procedure the doctor dilates your pupil and applies anesthetic drops to numb the eye. In cer-

Panretinal photocoagulation

Doctors generally treat proliferative diabetic retinopathy (PDR), in which many new blood vessels are forming, with panretinal, or scatter, photocoagulation. Using this technique, multiple laser burns hit the entire retina except for the macula. The treatment causes abnormal blood vessels to shrink and disappear over a wide area, reducing the chance of vitreous hemorrhage and traction retinal detachment.

Panretinal photocoagulation is usually done in two or more sessions. You may notice some loss of peripheral vision afterward. The procedure is a trade-off. Some of your side vision is sacrificed to save as much of your central vision as possible. You may also notice difficulties with your night vision and temporary blurring of your central vision. Panretinal photocoagulation doesn't always stop vision loss from diabetic retinopathy, even with repeated treatments.

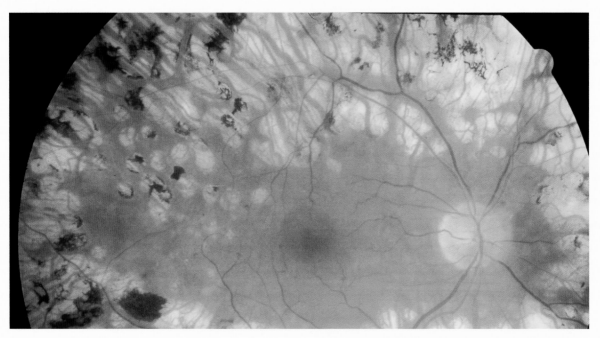

Panretinal photocoagulation covers most of the retina outside the macula. The mass of yellow spots on the image indicates where laser burns were applied to close off blood vessels and stop the leaking.

tain cases, the doctor will numb the eye completely by injecting an anesthetic around and behind the eye.

With your head resting in front of a slit lamp, a medical contact lens is placed on your cornea to help focus laser light onto the sections of the retina that will be treated. Fluorescein angiograms taken beforehand may serve as maps to show where the laser burns should be placed. During the procedure you may see bright flashes from the bursts of high-energy light.

To treat macular edema, the laser is focused on spots near the macula where blood vessels are leaking. The doctor makes "spot welds" to stop the leakage. If the leaks are small, the laser is applied to specific points where the leaks occur (focal laser treatment). If the leakage is widespread or diffuse, laser burns are applied in a grid pattern over a broad area (grid laser treatment).

After laser treatment, your vision will be blurry for about a day. You should be able to return home, but you won't be able to drive, so make sure to arrange for a ride. You may have some eye pain or a headache and be sensitive to light. An eye patch and over-the-counter pain relievers should help to ease the discomfort.

Immediately following laser surgery to treat macular edema, small spots — resulting from laser burns — may appear in your visual field. In addition, if you had blurred vision before surgery, you may not experience completely normal vision afterward.

Even when laser surgery is successful at sealing the leaks, new blood vessels may continue to grow and new leakage may occur. For this reason you'll have follow-up visits and, if necessary, additional laser treatments.

Vitrectomy

Sometimes, blood that has leaked into the vitreous from abnormal blood vessels will clear up on its own. But if the hemorrhage is massive and doesn't clear, the passage of light is blocked to your retina. A vitrectomy (vih-TREK-tuh-mee) may be required to remove the blockage.

This procedure to clear the vitreous also enables your eye doctor to examine your retina in greater detail, monitor symptoms of retinopathy and treat the condition, if needed.

In a vitrectomy, the surgeon makes small incisions in the eye and inserts several delicate instruments to remove the blood-filled vitreous. A vitreous cutter cuts the tissue and suctions it out, piece by piece. To maintain the shape and internal pressure of the eye, an infusion tube injects a balanced salt solution to replace the tissue that's being removed. A light probe illuminates the inside of the eye to help the surgeon to see better. The surgeon performs the procedure while looking through a microscope suspended over the eye. Removal of a dense

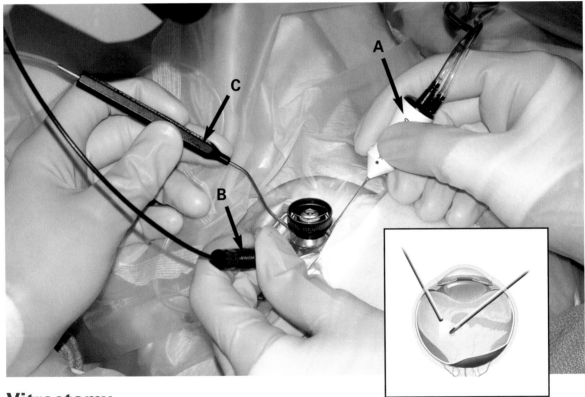

Vitrectomy

An external view of the procedure shows two instruments inserted into the eyeball: a vitreous cutter to cut tissue and suction it out (A) and a light probe for illumination (B). Even though the surgeon views the procedure through a surgical microscope, it's still necessary to hold a high-powered lens directly over the eye (C). The internal view (right) shows the cutter removing scar tissue and the light probe illuminating the eye.

hemorrhage in the vitreous generally re-establishes clear vision.

A vitrectomy can also be used to remove scar tissue, reducing the force (traction) that pulls the retina away from the underlying layers. This allows a detached retina to settle back and flatten out. Your doctor may decide not to operate on a retina detached by scar tissue if the detachment is located away from the macula and doesn't appear to be getting any worse.

Gas or silicone oil is placed in the eye to help keep the retina attached. The gas dissolves in about three to six weeks, depending on the type of gas used. Silicone oil is usually removed from the eye several weeks later.

During a vitrectomy, the surgeon may also perform panretinal photocoagulation to prevent the renewed growth of abnormal blood vessels.

Vitrectomy can be performed under local or general anesthesia. Your eye will likely be red, swollen and sensitive to light immediately afterward. For a short time, you'll need to wear an eye patch and apply medicated eyedrops to assist healing.

Full recovery may take weeks. When a vitrectomy is done for a massive vitreous hemorrhage, some blood may remain in the eye. Sometimes, fresh bleeding may occur. As the blood gradually dissipates, your sight should return to its former clarity.

Vision generally improves to previous levels in most people who receive surgery for a traction retinal detachment or vitreous hemorrhage. When the procedures fail to improve vision, it's usually because irreparable damage has occurred to the retina from diabetes. At other times it may be due to the complications of surgery, recurring bleeding from torn blood vessels or the development of neovascular glaucoma (see page 57).

Intravitreal injections

A new type of therapy under investigation for treating diabetic retinopathy involves injecting steroid medications directly into the vitreous (see pages 38-40). These medications have anti-inflammatory as well as anti-angiogenic properties, which means they may inhibit or stop abnormal blood vessels from growing in the eye. Having fewer of these fragile new blood vessels may reduce the amount of fluid and blood leaking into the retina and vitreous.

Several small studies using medications such as triamcinolone acetonide (Kenalog) and bevacizumab (Avastin) have produced positive results. Often, the participants in these studies have had long-term macular edema that has been unresponsive to surgical treatments.

Optical coherence tomography scans indicate that the macula can return to a normal thickness and contour following treatment. Visual acuity also generally stabilizes and, in some cases, improves — although not always to a degree that's desired.

More research is required before anti-angiogenic medications can become standard treatments for diabetic retinopathy. These studies will need to be larger and longer term in order to fully determine the medications' safety and efficacy. There also continue to be questions regarding the optimum dose and the frequency of additional treatment should macular edema recur. Several clinical trials sponsored by the National Eye Institute are under way that may resolve these concerns.

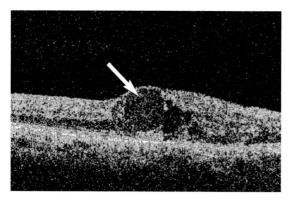 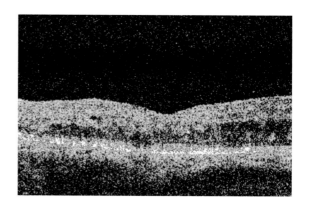

Anti-angiogenic therapy

In the optical coherence tomography (OCT) scan on the left, the macula is swollen from fluid accumulation in a cyst-like pocket (arrow). Following treatment with bevacizumab (Avastin), a later scan of the same eye (right) reveals that the edema has diminished and the macula has returned to normal contours.

Self-care

There are effective steps that you can take to help slow the progression of diabetic retinopathy.

Control your blood glucose. Tight control of your blood glucose (blood sugar) slows the onset and progression of retinopathy and lessens the need for surgery. Tight control means keeping your blood glucose levels as close to normal as possible. Ideally, this means levels between 90 and 130 milligrams of sugar per deciliter of blood (mg/dL) before meals and less than 180 mg/dL two hours after starting a meal.

Another measure of good control is a glycated hemoglobin level that's less than 7 percent. The glycated hemoglobin test (hemoglobin A1C test) measures how well you've controlled your blood glucose level over the previous two to three months.

Tight control isn't possible for everyone, including some older adults, young children and people with cardiovascular disease. Talk to your doctor or diabetes educator about a management plan that's best suited for

your personal goals. A management plan frequently involves:
* Taking regular doses of insulin or other medications
* Monitoring blood glucose levels
* Following a healthy-eating plan
* Getting regular exercise
* Maintaining a healthy weight

It may take some time before the benefits of lowering your blood glucose level are realized. And remember that better control reduces but doesn't eliminate your risk of developing retinopathy.

Be alert for vision changes. In addition to having an annual eye exam, be alert for any sudden changes in your vision. Have your eyes checked promptly if you experience vision changes that:
* Last more than a few days
* Aren't associated with changes in blood glucose levels
* Appear to be blurry, spotty or hazy
* Include eye pain, redness, floaters or light flashes

Keep your blood pressure down. Lowering your blood pressure level may help slow the progression of diabetic retinopathy. To reduce your blood pressure, you may need to take medications or make certain lifestyle changes.

Stop smoking. Smoking is especially harmful for people with diabetes and high blood pressure because the habit helps clog or block blood circulation.

Limit alcohol. Drinking more than moderate amounts of alcohol can increase your blood pressure and interfere with the medications you're taking. Alcohol also increases the risk of low blood glucose levels.

Control stress. Stress can cause wide swings in blood pressure and blood glucose levels. Stress also may affect your ability to control blood glucose, for example, making you too busy or preoccupied to exercise or eat a good meal. Don't hesitate to seek help from a counselor, therapist or support group. Relaxation techniques such as meditation also may be helpful.

Maintain a healthy weight. Your weight and your blood pressure and blood glucose levels tend to go hand in hand. When your weight increases, your blood pressure and blood glucose often do, as well. And being overweight is a key risk factor for diabetes. As Americans become increasingly overweight, controlling weight has become a major challenge in preventing and treating high blood pressure and diabetes.

Exercise. Regular physical activity helps you control diabetes by reducing the amount of glucose in your bloodstream. Physical activity is also a key factor for managing many other chronic conditions, including high blood pressure.

Chapter 4

Retinal detachment

and other retinal disorders

Previous chapters have described two major diseases that damage the retina: macular degeneration and diabetic retinopathy. This chapter examines other conditions that affect the retina and optic nerve, especially retinal detachment.

The retina, you'll recall, is a thin, layer of tissue that converts light into electric signals (see pages 22-23). Attached to the back of the retina is the optic nerve, a bundle of nerve fibers that serves as a superhighway along which the signals race back and forth between the eye and the brain.

This chapter begins by describing basic changes to the retina and optic nerve that occur in almost everyone's eyes over time. Later in the chapter, the discussion turns to lesser known conditions that can develop at the back of your eye.

While some of the changes described in this chapter may seem to have little impact on your vision, they can also be warning signs of more serious developments. Other changes may cause severe vision loss or blindness, if left untreated. The key is being alert to the signs and symptoms.

Floaters and flashes

The large internal cavity of your eye is filled with a clear substance called the vitreous. Eye floaters are small bits of debris floating in the vitreous. They may appear as spots, hairs or bits of string that dart into your field of vision. Floaters are most noticeable in bright light, for example, when you're outside on a sunny day or if you're in a room with white walls.

Eye floaters are due to age-related alterations to the vitreous. Over time, the vitreous changes in consistency and partially liquifies — a process that causes it to shrink and pull away from the interior surface of the eyeball. This development is called posterior vitreous detachment (PVD), or vitreous collapse.

According to one estimate, about 90 percent of people over age 40 experience this change to some extent. Other risk factors for vitreous collapse include nearsightedness, eye trauma, inflammation, diseases such as diabetic retinopathy, and complications from cataract surgery.

Vitreous collapse generally doesn't cause vision loss and no treatment may be necessary. But the shrinking and sagging causes the vitreous to become more fibrous and stringy. When floaters appear in your visual field, what you're seeing are the shadows these strings cast on the retina. Although bothersome, the floaters generally aren't a serious problem.

You may also see flashes of sparkling lights (photopsia) in your peripheral

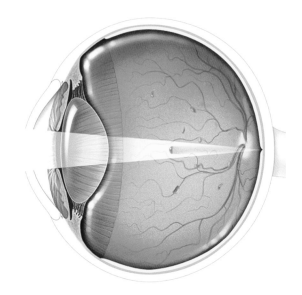

Floaters

Tiny pieces of debris floating in the vitreous block some of the light passing through the eye, casting shadows on the retina and obstructing vision.

vision when your eyes are closed or if you're in a darkened room. This phenomenon generally lasts only a few seconds. The flashes occur because some of the fibers in the vitreous are still attached to the retina and pull on the retinal surface as the vitreous sags. The flashes appear in your side vision because the fibers tend to be more firmly attached to the retina around its periphery.

Floaters generally increase in number gradually. In rare instances, the number and size of the floaters may interfere with your central vision. In such cases, a doctor may recommend surgical removal of the floating debris with a vitrectomy (see pages 63-65). However, this surgery carries risks and it may not remove all floaters.

There are times when floaters can be a much greater concern. See your ophthalmologist immediately if you notice a sudden onset of floaters or a significant increase in the number of floaters — especially if they're associated with photopsia or hazy vision. The sudden onset of floaters or a large increase in their numbers could be the sign of a potentially serious eye disorder, such as a retinal tear or retinal detachment.

Macular pucker

When the vitreous sags and tugs on the retina, there often can be microscopic damage to the retinal surface. As part of the healing process, scar tissue may form around the damaged area. Typically, the scar tissue begins to shrink over time, causing the retina to wrinkle, or pucker.

A small amount of scar tissue on the retinal surface generally has little effect on vision. But when enough scar tissue forms on the macula, causing a pucker, vision may become blurred or distorted. You may have difficulty seeing fine detail, or part of your central vision may be clouded.

The symptoms of a macular pucker — blurriness and distortion — are often mild and require no treatment. People simply adjust to the change. If the symptoms are more severe, a vitrectomy may be necessary to remove the scar tissue.

Once a macular pucker has formed, vision usually stabilizes after the initial change and doesn't progressively worsen. Usually just one eye is affected, but puckers may occur in both eyes. A pucker generally doesn't cause a tear or hole to form in the macular surface.

Retinal tear and macular hole

When the pull of a sagging vitreous becomes strong enough, the retina may tear, forming a small, jagged flap on its surface. Most tears occur along the periphery of the retina, where fibers in the vitreous are more firmly attached and can't separate without hard tugging.

Retinal tears and holes are a common result of aging and usually occur in people over age 60. These tiny breaks are usually caused by the shrinking vitreous, but retinal holes may also develop where the retina has simply become thin. Other causes of retinal tears and holes include nearsighted-ness and eye trauma.

When a hole forms on the macula, the consequences are more noticeable because the macula is responsible for central vision (see picture on page 46). Signs and symptoms develop

gradually. In the early stages, there may be blurred vision — comparable to the vision changes from a macular pucker. However, the two are very different conditions.

Some small retinal holes require no treatment and seal themselves as the tissue heals. In other cases, fluid from the vitreous seeps through the tear and pools under the surface, causing surrounding sections of the retina to detach from the underlying layer. This can lead to severe vision loss.

Treatment for retinal tears

If the retina hasn't detached from the underlying layer around the tear,

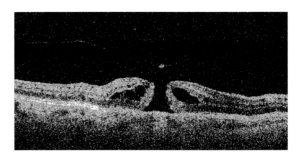

Macular hole

A cross section of the retina on this optical coherence tomography scan reveals a large macular hole, which can blur vision and cause visual distortions.

your eye surgeon may suggest one of two procedures: photocoagulation or cryopexy. With either procedure, healing of the tear typically takes from 10 to 14 days.

Photocoagulation. In this procedure, a surgeon uses a laser beam to make burns around the retinal tear (see pages 36-37). The burns cause scarring, which usually welds the retina to the underlying tissue. This procedure requires no surgical incision, and causes less irritation to the eye than does cryopexy.

Cryopexy. With this procedure, the surgeon uses intense cold to freeze tissue around the retinal tear. After a local anesthetic has numbed your eye, a freezing probe is applied to the outer surface of the eye directly over the retinal defect. The freezing produces an inflammation that causes scarring, again welding the retina to the underlying tissue, much like with photocoagulation.

Cryopexy (KRI-o-pek-see) is used when the tears are more difficult to reach with a laser, generally along the retinal periphery. Your eye may be red and swollen for some time after the procedure.

Retinal detachment

Retinal detachment is a medical emergency, and timing is critical when it comes to treatment. Unless the detached retina is promptly re-attached surgically, this condition can cause permanent vision loss or blindness in the affected eye.

Retinal detachment occurs when fluid leaking through a tear or break causes part of the retina to peel away from underlying layers — the retinal pigment epithelium and the choroid. As liquid collects under the retina from continued leakage, the detachment expands, like wallpaper slowly peeling off a wall. Areas where the retina is detached can no longer function, and vision begins to blur.

Not all tears and holes in the retina lead to retinal detachment. Sometimes the retinal layer surrounding these defects remains relatively well attached. But more often, leakage from the vitreous causes separation.

Detachment that goes undetected and untreated can eventually involve

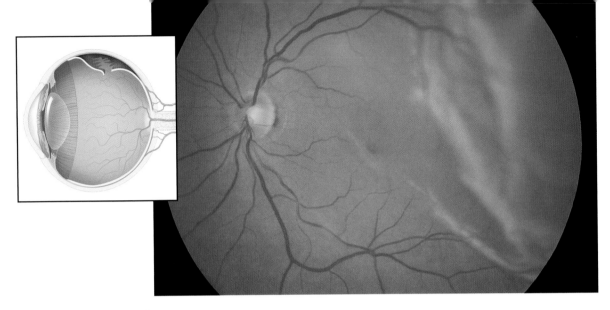

Retinal detachment

A section of the retina that has pulled away from the inside back wall of the eye appears gray and folded on this color fundus photograph. Most retinal detachments occur in the upper half of the eyeball due to the effects of gravity on the sagging vitreous (see inset).

the entire retina. Typically, scar tissue forms over the retinal surface and the retina will become stiff. At this stage — even if extensive surgery is performed — it's unlikely you'll regain the vision you had in the eye before the detachment occurred.

Other, less common causes of retinal detachment include traction from scar tissue on the retinal surface, as what may occur in individuals with diabetes. Sometimes, retinal detachment may occur without a retinal break. This is known as serous retinal detachment. The condition can stem from the leakage of fluid under the

retina due to trauma, a tumor or an inflammatory condition.

Signs and symptoms

Retinal detachment is painless, but other warning signs typically appear before the detachment occurs. The signs often include:

- The sudden appearance of many floaters — when your retina tears, pigment may be released into the vitreous, or small blood vessels may be broken and leak blood that seeps into the vitreous
- Sudden flashes of light in one or both eyes

- A shadow or curtain falls over a portion of your visual field
- A sudden blurriness in your vision — because most tears occur along the periphery of the retina, the blurring may first be noticeable in your peripheral vision

If you experience any of these signs or symptoms, seek urgent evaluation by an ophthalmologist. Although floaters or flashes usually don't indicate a serious problem, if they're caused by a retinal detachment, prompt treatment is critical to preserve your vision.

Unfortunately, many people don't appreciate the urgency of the warning signs, and they tend to delay seeing an eye doctor in the hope that the symptoms will disappear. In some cases, the symptoms will temporarily diminish only to be followed by a sudden loss of vision over the next few days or weeks, caused by advanced retinal detachment.

Retinal detachment can't always be successfully repaired with surgery, and vision loss may become permanent. See your doctor as soon as you notice that something isn't right with your vision.

Risk factors

Your risk of developing a detached retina generally increases with age, simply because the vitreous changes as you grow older. A detached retina is more common among men than women. You're also at greater risk if any of these factors apply to you:

- Previous retinal detachment in one eye
- Family history of retinal detachment
- Extreme nearsightedness
- Previous eye surgery, such as cataract removal
- Previous severe eye injury or eye trauma
- Weak areas along the periphery of your retina

An ophthalmologist can determine if you have a retinal detachment by carefully examining the retina with an ophthalmoscope, which allows a doctor to view the inside of your eyes in great detail.

Treatment

Surgery is the only effective therapy for a retinal detachment, and time is critical in determining how to proceed. If a tear or hole can be treated before detachment begins, or if a retinal detachment is treated before the macula is affected, you'll likely retain much of your vision. It's best if surgery can be performed within days of the diagnosis.

Three different surgical procedures are commonly used by doctors to repair a detached retina: pneumatic retinopexy, scleral buckling and vit-rectomy. The first two procedures are performed with cryopexy (see page 73). Vitrectomy may be required to clear a massive vitreous hemorrhage or to remove scar tissue before the retina is reattached.

The purposes of treatment are to reseal the tear and stop the leakage of fluid, reduce the tug of a shrinking vitreous, and reattach the loosened

Vitreous hemorrhage and retinal detachment

A vitreous hemorrhage occurs when blood spills into the vitreous cavity from torn blood vessels around a retinal tear. Treating a retinal detachment in the presence of a vitreous hemorrhage can be difficult because blood clouds the vitreous and prevents the surgeon from getting a clear view of the retina. When this happens, the surgeon uses ultrasonography to locate the tear and assess the damage.

Ultrasonography is a painless test that sends sound waves through the clouded vitreous to bounce off the retina (see page 48). The returning sound waves are captured in a digital image that allows the doctor to determine the condition of the retina and other structures inside the eye. If a retinal detachment is found, a vitrectomy may be required to remove blood from the vitreous before the surgeon can repair the retina.

In this situation you're at high risk of developing scar tissue in the vitreous and on the retina, a condition called proliferative vitreoretinopathy. The condition occurs when scar tissue folds or puckers the retina, preventing the retina from being reattached by standard surgical means alone.

portion of the retina to the back of the eyeball. The severity and complexity of your condition will determine which treatment your eye surgeon recommends.

Pneumatic retinopexy. This surgical procedure is used for an uncomplicated detachment when the tear is located in the upper half of the retina. It's usually done on an outpatient basis under local anesthesia.

First, the surgeon performs cryopexy to seal the retinal tear. Then he or she withdraws a small amount of fluid from the anterior chamber to soften the eye. Next, the surgeon injects a bubble of expandable gas into the vitreous cavity. Over the next several days, the gas bubble expands, pushing against the detached area. With no new fluid passing through the retinal tear, fluid that had previously collected under the retina is absorbed, and the retina reattaches itself to the back of the eye.

After surgery, you may have to hold your head in an upright or sideways position for a few days to make sure the gas bubble seals around the retinal tear. It takes several weeks for the bubble to disappear completely. Until the gas is gone from your eye, you have to avoid lying or sleeping on your back. This keeps the bubble away from your lens and reduces the risk of cataract formation or a sudden pressure increase in your eye.

During recovery, you can't travel by airplane or be at a high altitude because a sudden drop in pressure would cause the gas bubble to expand rapidly, resulting in dangerously high eye pressure. Your surgeon can advise you on when the danger has passed.

The success rate of pneumatic retinopexy isn't as good as that of scleral buckling. However, it can prevent a trip to the operating room and the need for incisional surgery.

Complications may include:
- Recurring retinal detachment
- Excessive scar tissue formation
- Cataracts
- Glaucoma (due to an increase in pressure from the gas bubble)
- Gas collecting under the retina
- Infection

These complications are rare, but if they do occur and go untreated, they can cause severe loss of vision.

Recurrent retinal detachment can usually be repaired with scleral buckling or vitrectomy.

Scleral buckling. A primary goal of this procedure is to slightly reduce the circumference of the eyeball, which helps to reattach the retina and to relieve some of the tension on the retina caused by the shrinking vitreous. This procedure is usually performed in an operating room under local or general anesthesia and often on an outpatient basis.

First, the surgeon treats the retinal tears with cryopexy. Then he or she indents (buckles) the sclera over the affected area by pressing on the eyeball with a piece of silicone. The silicone material is either a soft sponge or a solid piece. Gentle external pressure from the buckle promotes healing by helping to close the separation between the retina and underlying layers. Also by reducing the size of the eyeball, the buckle prevents or reduces further pulling and tugging by the vitreous.

If you have a single tear, the buckle may be placed directly over the detached area. If you have several tears or an extensive detachment, the surgeon may create an encircling scleral buckle around the entire circumference of the eye. The buckle is stitched to the outer surface of the sclera. Before tying the sutures holding the buckle in place, the surgeon may make a small cut in the sclera to drain fluid that has collected under the detached retina. Once the incision heals, there is little evidence of the

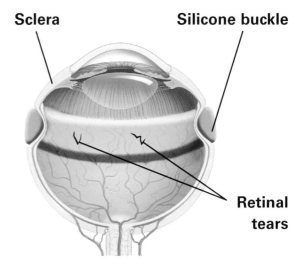

Sclera   Silicone buckle

Retinal tears

Encircling scleral buckle

Silicone material stitched to the outside of the eye indents or "buckles" the sclera, making the eyeball smaller. A smaller circumference assists the healing process by pushing the choroid against the detached retina. It also reduces the amount of traction placed on the retina by a shrinking vitreous.

operation, and the buckle remains in place for the rest of your life. Some surgeons may choose a temporary buckle for simple retinal detachments, using a small rubber balloon that's inflated and later removed.

Scleral buckling is generally successful with one operation but a reattached retina doesn't guarantee that you'll have normal vision. How well you see after surgery depends in part on how much of the retina was affected by the detachment and for how long. Your sight isn't likely to return to normal if the macula was ever detached. Even if the macula wasn't affected and scleral buckling successfully repairs the retinal tear, you have a 10 percent chance of losing some vision due to wrinkling or puckering of the macula.

If the first operation fails, your doctor may attempt to reattach the retina with one or more additional operations. Additional surgery increases the rate of successful reattachment.

Sometimes, after the procedure, the retina fails to firmly reattach. This is often due to scar tissue that had formed on the retinal surface before the operation. Scar tissue that forms after the operation may cause the retina to separate once again after having been attached. If this happens, it's usually within the first couple of months after surgery. Surgery to remove the scar tissue may again become necessary.

Complications from scleral buckling occur infrequently but may result in the loss of some or all vision in the eye or, in rare instances, the loss of the eye. The complications may include:

- Bleeding under the retina or into the vitreous cavity. This can occur inadvertently while subretinal fluid is being drained or when a buckle suture perforates the sclera and enters the eye.
- Increased pressure inside the eye (glaucoma). This is due to a swelling of the choroid and narrowing of the angle in the anterior chamber.
- Double vision (diplopia). This is a common side effect of scleral buckles. It occurs because the buckle passes underneath the eye muscles. The condition is usually temporary and may require corrective glasses with prisms. Occasionally, surgery is needed to remove the buckle or reposition the eye muscles.

Vitrectomy. Sometimes, bleeding or inflammation clouds the vitreous and blocks the surgeon's view of the detached retina. In other cases, scar tissue makes it impossible to repair a retinal detachment. In these situations, a procedure called vitrectomy may be required (see pages 63-65). Scleral buckling also may be included in the surgery.

Many people who have a vitrectomy will have a gas or silicone oil bubble placed in the eye. The bubble assists healing by holding the retina in place. Gas bubbles are absorbed into the body over time but an oil bubble remains in the eye until it's surgically removed. As long as the bubble is in your eye, you'll need to follow the same precautions as are necessary following pneumatic retinopexy.

After surgery. Expect your eye to be red, swollen, watery and slightly sore for up to a month after any of the surgical procedures just described. Wearing an eye patch may provide some temporary relief. Your doctor may also prescribe antibacterial or dilating eyedrops to help the healing process. Severe pain is unlikely, but if it should occur, contact your surgeon immediately for treatment.

It'll take about eight to 10 weeks for your eye to heal fully. You should avoid strenuous activities during this time. As your vision stabilizes, your doctor can help determine if you need corrective lenses or adjustments to an existing prescription. Vision may take many months to improve after surgery to repair a complicated retinal detachment. Some people don't recover any lost vision.

Retinal blood vessel blockage

Intricate networks of tiny arteries and veins are located in the retina. The arteries and veins are close together, sometimes crossing over and intertwining with each other. Both networks connect to major blood vessels — the central retinal artery and the central retinal vein — that enter the eyeball through the optic nerve.

Sometimes, these arteries and veins can become blocked, a condition known as retinal vessel occlusion. The condition is common in older adults and can result in reduced vision or vision loss.

A variety of factors can obstruct blood vessels, such as a blood clot or the accumulation of fatty deposits (plaques). A blockage can also result from the collapse of vessel walls or from outside pressure that compresses the walls. When a retinal artery is obstructed, oxygen-rich blood is unable to nourish the retina. When a retinal vein is obstructed, blood is unable to leave the retina, causing the retina to swell.

The extent of vision loss that accompanies this condition is dependent on several factors, including how much time has elapsed before treatment begins, the location of the blockage and the presence of swelling.

There are four types of retinal vessel blockages:

Branch retinal vein occlusion (BRVO). Blockage causes blood to back up in the capillary network and pressure to build within the retina. The increased pressure can lead to leakage and bleeding from the capillaries and swelling (edema) in the macula, blurring vision or causing "blind spots." BRVO is the second most common circulatory disorder of the retina after diabetic retinopathy.

Grid laser photocoagulation may be used to treat the edema by placing a few laser spots in a grid pattern on the macula. Other ways of treating edema include injecting a steroid or anti-angiogenic agent into the eye.

A potential complication of BRVO is the growth of new blood vessels on the optic nerve, retina or iris. If left untreated, these vessels may hemorrhage into the vitreous. Blood vessel growth on the iris may cause neovascular glaucoma accompanied by a profound, irreversible loss of vision. Panretinal laser treatment may be used to halt the new vessel growth.

Central retinal vein occlusion (CRVO). Blockage occurs in the large retinal vein, which collects all of the blood that has passed through the capillaries. CRVO causes branch veins to engorge and the retina surrounding the optic nerve to swell. Vision loss may be mild to severe. As with BRVO, vision loss occurs from poor blood supply to the retina and leakage from capillaries, causing macular edema. Unlike BRVO, grid laser photocoagulation for edema isn't effective, and the condition must be treated with injections of a steroid or anti-angiogenic agent into the eye.

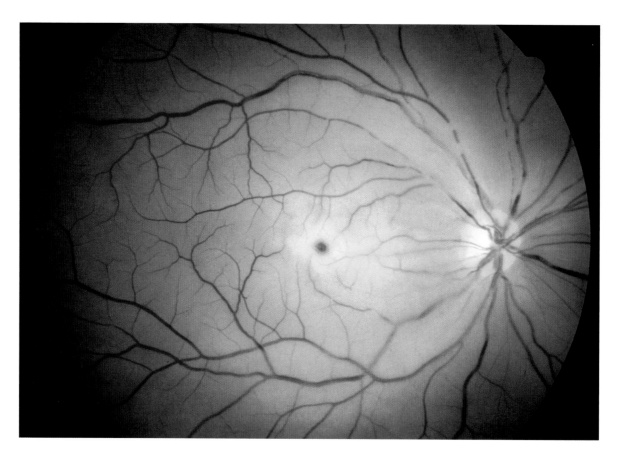

Central retinal artery occlusion

The pale retina on this color fundus photograph is a result of blockage in the central retinal artery that prevents sufficient blood flow to the eye.

The growth of new blood vessels on the optic nerve, retina or iris may also occur with CRVO and may be treated with the panretinal laser procedure.

Branch retinal artery occlusion (BRAO). Blockage occurs in one of the small branch arteries, limiting blood supply to the retina. The blockage is often the result of a blood clot or abnormal particle (embolus) that has become lodged in a small vessel. Partial vision loss — sometimes of central vision — that happens abruptly is usually the earliest indication of this problem.

Although there's currently no proven treatment to regain lost vision, it's important to find out why BRAO has occurred. Risk factors include high blood pressure, high cholesterol, abnormal clotting, diabetes, coronary artery disease and narrowing of the carotid artery. The most common cause of BRAO is an embolus. Other causes include inflammation of the blood vessels (vasculitis) or the eye (uveitis) and clotting abnormalities.

Central retinal artery occlusion (CRAO). Blockage of the main retinal artery significantly obstructs blood flow to the retina (see photograph on page 82). The condition is sometimes referred to as a "stroke" of the eye and generally results in sudden, profound vision loss. The causes and risk factors of CRAO are similar to those of BRAO. Neovascular glaucoma is a potential complication.

Experimental treatments at present are aimed at dislodging the obstruction from the vessel. They include ocular massage, removal of aqueous humor from the eye and inhaling an oxygen and carbon dioxide mixture. Chances of improved vision are best if treatment occurs less than 24 hours from the onset of symptoms.

Disorders of the optic nerve

The optic nerve is the vital pathway in which the eye communicates with the brain. It's analogous to the high-speed fiber-optic cable that links homes with television and Internet service. Problems with the optic nerve may interfere with signal transmission and cause vision loss.

Optic neuritis

Optic neuritis is an inflammation of the optic nerve anywhere along its path. The inflammation may stem from a viral illness or certain autoimmune diseases, such as multiple sclerosis. Frequently, the cause of optic neuritis is unknown.

When the condition affects the optic disk, it's known as papillitis. When the inflammation occurs in the portion of the optic nerve behind the eye, it's known as retrobulbar neuritis.

When the optic nerve swells, it blocks signals to the brain. The result is a gradual or sudden loss of vision in one or both eyes. With retrobulbar neuritis, eye movement may be painful. In the case of papillitis, loss of vision is the only symptom.

In most cases, optic neuritis disappears within two to eight weeks without treatment, and vision returns to normal. An MRI scan of the brain is often done to determine the risk of multiple sclerosis. If you're at high risk, your doctor may administer an intravenous steroid or interferon beta-1a to reduce the risk of multiple sclerosis and improve the prognosis.

Papilledema

Papilledema (pap-il-uh-DEE-muh) is a swelling of the optic disk caused by an elevated pressure within the skull. The abnormal high pressure may be caused by a tumor, abscess, hemorrhage or infection in the brain. Vision usually isn't affected in the early stages of papilledema. As the condition progresses, symptoms such as blurred vision may occur for a few seconds, then disappear. Treatment of papilledema will depend on what is the cause — for example, surgery to remove a tumor or antibiotics to fight infection. The prognosis is usually good if the intracranial pressure can be controlled.

Ischemic optic neuropathy

Ischemic optic neuropathy is a painless swelling of the optic nerve due to the loss of blood supply. This may lead to impaired function or death of nerve cells. The degree of vision loss varies but may become severe and permanent. It can occur over minutes and hours, or it may develop gradually over several days. Both eyes can be involved.

The condition most often develops in adults age 50 and older and may be associated with an underlying chronic condition such as high blood pressure, atherosclerosis or diabetes. It may also result from inflammation of the arteries in the scalp and head (temporal arteritis).

Treatment involves controlling certain factors that affect blood supply to the optic nerve, such as blood pressure and cholesterol. Corticosteroid medications may be administered if the condition is a result of temporal arteritis — to help prevent vision loss in the second eye.

Chapter 5

Glaucoma

Glaucoma is sometimes called the silent thief. That's because the most common form of glaucoma develops with no warning signs. Many people aren't even aware they have a problem until their vision is extensively damaged. Glaucoma is a serious vision threat. It's the second most common cause of vision loss in the United States, after age-related macular degeneration.

Actually, glaucoma is not one disease but a group of them. The feature they have in common is damage to the optic nerve, which carries signals from the eye to the brain. The condition is usually accompanied by abnormally high pressure within the eye.

As the optic nerve deteriorates, blind spots develop in your visual field, usually starting with your side (peripheral) vision. The exact cause of glaucoma isn't known, but a number of factors may be involved, including inflammation and vascular, mechanical and even neurotransmitter problems.

Fortunately, only a small percentage of people with glaucoma ever lose their sight completely. That's because medical advances have made it easier to treat the disease. If detected early, glaucoma need not cause even moderate vision loss. But having glaucoma does require regular monitoring and treatment for the rest of your life.

Damaged cells

Vision loss in glaucoma results from disrupted communication between the eye and the brain due to damaged cells in the optic nerve. It's unclear why, but when optic nerve cells are damaged, they inevitably die rather than stabilize or repair themselves. Researchers are trying to find out why this takes place.

Doctors have debated for many years about how damage to the optic nerve occurs. One theory holds that abnormal eye pressure causes structural damage in the optic nerve and ultimately death to the nerve fibers. Another theory suggests that the nerve fibers die when small blood vessels that feed the optic nerve become blocked or obstructed due to the increased pressure, starving the cells.

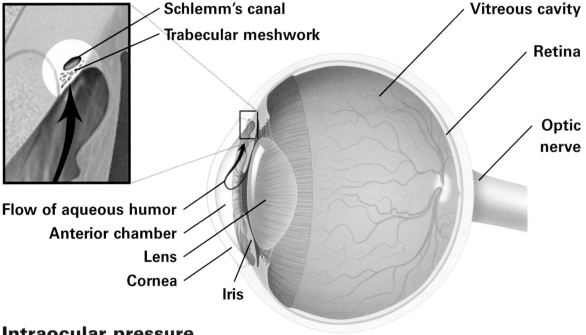

Schlemm's canal
Trabecular meshwork
Vitreous cavity
Retina
Optic nerve
Flow of aqueous humor
Anterior chamber
Lens
Cornea
Iris

Intraocular pressure

The flow of aqueous humor through the anterior chamber at the front of the eye plays a role in intraocular pressure. Aqueous humor exits the eye where the iris and cornea meet (see inset). The fluid filters through the trabecular meshwork before passing into an open channel called Schlemm's canal. Increased resistance to flow at the trabecular meshwork can increase pressure within the eye.

Understanding eye pressure

Internal eye pressure, called intraocular pressure (IOP), allows the eye to hold its shape and function properly. Think of IOP as air in a balloon — the right amount of air pressure keeps the balloon round and taut, but too much pressure can cause problems.

Abnormally high eye pressure puts you at a greatly increased risk of glaucoma. However, high intraocular pressure doesn't mean that you have glaucoma. Some people seem better able to tolerate a higher IOP than do others, without suffering damage to the optic nerve. In addition, you can develop glaucoma even if your eye pressure is within the range of what's considered normal — between 10 and 22 millimeters of mercury (mm Hg). So eye pressure may only be a single contributing factor in the process.

To better understand eye pressure, it's helpful to know more about the mechanisms that help regulate IOP and what may cause pressure to change. An increase in eye pressure is influenced by the flow of aqueous humor, a fluid that circulates through your eye's anterior chamber.

Aqueous humor is produced within the eye and circulates around the lens and cornea before draining out of the eye (see the illustration on page 86). This continuous flow nourishes the eye and removes unwanted debris.

Aqueous humor exits the eye through a sieve-like drainage system located at the angle where the iris and the cornea meet. Here the fluid passes through spongy tissue known as the trabecular meshwork. Fluid then drains into an open channel called Schlemm's canal and eventually is absorbed into the body's bloodstream. Your eye produces aqueous humor at about the same rate as the fluid drains.

When the drainage system doesn't function properly — for example, if the trabecular meshwork becomes clogged — drainage of aqueous humor is obstructed. This increased resistance raises pressure within the eye. Increased resistance is almost always the cause of elevated IOP.

There are occasions when the trabecular meshwork becomes completely blocked. The blockage causes a rapid increase in eye pressure, an emergency situation.

Types

There are several types of glaucoma. The differences between the various types have to do with what's causing the blockage that results in increased resistance to aqueous humor draining out of the eye.

Primary open-angle

Primary open-angle glaucoma, also known as chronic open-angle glaucoma, is the most common form of the disease. Although the angle formed by the cornea and the iris remains open, a resistance develops to the aqueous humor draining through the trabecular meshwork. This resistance causes a gradual buildup of pressure within the eye. Damage to the optic nerve is slow and painless. A large part of your vision can be lost before you're even aware of a problem.

The cause of primary open-angle glaucoma remains unknown. It may be age-related — the aqueous humor drains less efficiently as you grow older. But then, not all older adults get this form of glaucoma. About 8 percent of Americans older than age 70 have elevated eye pressure. The

condition may be genetic and is more common in individuals who have relatives with the disease.

Angle-closure

Angle-closure glaucoma, also called closed-angle glaucoma, occurs when the sharp angle formed by the cornea and the iris narrows. This angle forms a passage for the aqueous humor to reach the trabecular meshwork and drain out of the eye. When the channel narrows, resistance to aqueous humor flowing through the passage increases and pressure within the eye goes up. This gradual development is known as chronic angle-closure glaucoma.

Sometimes, the angle between the cornea and iris can close off completely, blocking aqueous humor from reaching the trabecular meshwork. This causes the sudden onset of acute angle-closure glaucoma, which is a medical emergency.

Angle-closure glaucoma is less common than is open-angle glaucoma. Many people who develop the acute form have always had a very narrow drainage angle, which may be an abnormality from birth. Angle-

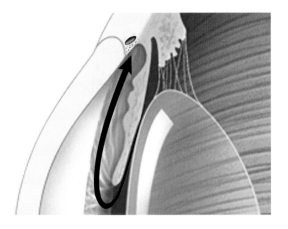

Open-angle glaucoma

Blockage of the trabecular meshwork resists the drainage of aqueous humor out of the eye, increasing intraocular pressure.

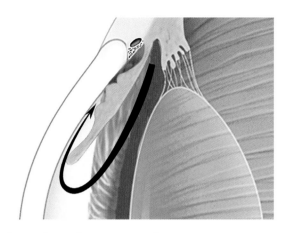

Angle-closure glaucoma

With the acute form, the angle formed by the cornea and the iris closes completely, preventing aqueous humor from draining out of the eye. This leads to a sudden, rapid increase in intraocular pressure.

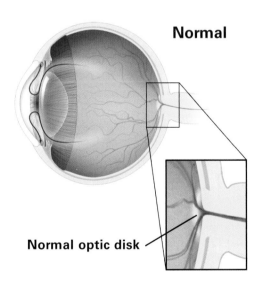

Normal

Normal optic disk

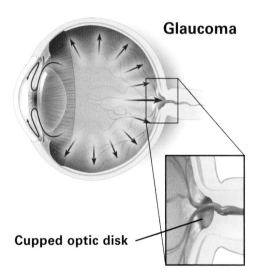

Glaucoma

Cupped optic disk

Damage to the optic disk

Evidence of glaucoma includes damaged nerve fibers in the optic nerve, causing the optic disk to appear "cupped" or excavated (see also the photo on page 95).

closure glaucoma is more common among farsighted people, who tend to have smaller eyes. Normal aging also may cause the angle to narrow. As you get older, your lens becomes larger, pushing the iris forward and narrowing the angle.

Sometimes, if the pupils are dilated in a person whose eyes already have a narrow drainage angle, the angle may close completely, causing a sudden increase in eye pressure. Certain factors that can cause your pupils to dilate include:

- Darkness or dim light
- Stress or excitement
- Certain medications, including antihistamines, tricyclic antidepressants and eyedrops used to dilate your pupils. Dilating eyedrops may not cause the angle to close until several hours after the drops are put in.

Acute angle-closure glaucoma is a medical emergency that requires immediate medical treatment. It can cause vision loss within hours of its onset, and without treatment blindness can develop in the eye in as little as one or two days. Although an acute attack often affects only one eye, the other eye is at risk of attack.

Secondary

Glaucoma is referred to as secondary when it's a complication of another medical condition. (By contrast, glaucoma is known as a primary condition if the cause is unknown.) Secondary glaucoma may stem from a variety of diseases, medications, physical injuries or trauma, and eye inflammation or abnormalities. Infrequently, eye surgery can cause secondary glaucoma. Examples of secondary glaucoma include pseudoexfoliative glaucoma, which occurs when small particles produced in the eye accumulate and block the trabecular meshwork, and neovascular glaucoma, which is associated with diabetes (see page 57).

Low-tension

Low-tension glaucoma is a poorly understood, though not uncommon, form of the disease. In this form, eye pressure stays within what's considered a normal range but the optic nerve is damaged nevertheless. Why this happens is unknown, although some experts believe that people with low-tension glaucoma may have an abnormally fragile optic nerve or a reduced blood supply to the optic nerve, caused by a condition such as atherosclerosis. Under these circumstances, even normal pressure on the optic nerve would be enough to cause damage.

Signs and symptoms

Primary open-angle glaucoma and chronic angle-closure glaucoma develop with few or no symptoms until they're at an advanced stage. As damage to the optic nerve continues, you lose more and more of your peripheral vision. You'll have trouble seeing objects off to the side or out of the corner of your eye. Over time, it may start to feel like you're looking through a tunnel.

These types of glaucoma usually affect both eyes, although at first you may have vision loss in just one eye. Other symptoms include:
- Sensitivity to light and glare
- Trouble differentiating between varying shades of light and dark
- Trouble with night vision

Acute angle-closure glaucoma develops suddenly in response to a rapid rise in eye pressure. An attack often happens in the evening or in a room when the light is dim and your

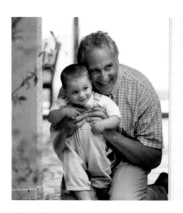 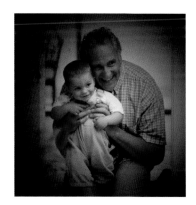 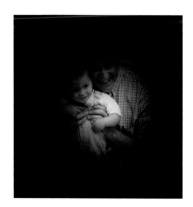

Vision with glaucoma

The gradual loss of peripheral vision is shown in this sequence from a normal visual field (left) to early-stage glaucoma (center) to advanced-stage glaucoma (right). Very often, you're unaware of this gradual narrowing of your visual field until an advanced stage.

pupils have become dilated. Signs and symptoms include:

- Blurred vision
- Halos around lights
- Reddening of the eye
- Severe headache or eye pain
- Nausea and vomiting

If any of these signs or symptoms occurs, get immediate medical attention. Permanent vision loss can occur within hours of the attack.

Signs and symptoms of secondary glaucoma will vary, depending on what's causing the glaucoma and whether the drainage angle remains open or closed.

Risk factors

If your intraocular pressure is higher than what's considered normal, you're at increased risk of developing glaucoma, although not everyone with elevated pressure develops the disease. This makes it difficult to predict who will get glaucoma. Other factors are also known to increase your risk. Because chronic forms of glaucoma can destroy vision before symptoms become apparent, it's

important to be aware of the following risk factors:

Age. Open-angle glaucoma is rare before age 40. Everyone older than 60 is at increased risk of glaucoma. For blacks, however, the increased risk develops earlier, after age 40.

Race. In the United States, blacks have a much higher risk of glaucoma

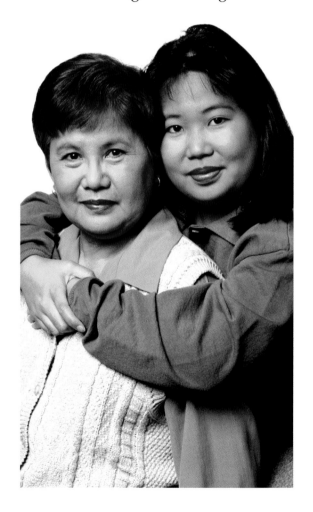

than do whites, and they're much more likely to experience permanent blindness as a result. Hispanics also face a higher risk. Asians are at a higher risk of angle-closure glaucoma and Japanese are more prone to low-tension glaucoma. The reasons for these difference aren't clear.

Family history. If there's a member in your immediate family who has glaucoma, you have a much greater risk of developing the disease. This suggests a genetic link, meaning there's a defect in one or more genes that may cause certain individuals to be more susceptible to disease.

Medical conditions. Diabetes, high blood pressure, heart disease and hypothyroidism can increase your risk of developing glaucoma. Other risk factors include vascular problems such as stroke and Raynaud's disease, as well as eye inflammation, such as chronic uveitis and iritis. Previous eye surgery may trigger secondary glaucoma.

Physical injuries. Severe trauma, such as being hit in the eye, can result in increased eye pressure. Injury can also dislocate the lens, closing the drainage angle.

Nearsightedness. Being nearsighted, which means that objects in the distance look fuzzy without glasses or contacts, increases the risk of developing open-angle glaucoma.

Prolonged corticosteroid use. Using corticosteroids for prolonged periods of time appears to put you at risk of developing secondary glaucoma.

Eye abnormalities. Structural abnormalities of the eye can lead to secondary glaucoma.

Screening and diagnosis

Routine eye exams are the key to detecting glaucoma early enough for successful treatment. Don't wait for problems of any kind to occur. If you have one or more risk factors for glaucoma, talk to your doctor about scheduling regular appointments.

It's best to have an eye checkup every two to four years after age 40 and every one to two years after age 65. If you're at increased risk, your doctor may recommend more frequent monitoring. Because blacks have a much higher risk of glaucoma, screening should begin every three to five years from age 20 to 29, and every two to four years after age 30.

In addition, be alert for signs and symptoms of an acute angle-closure glaucoma attack, such as a severe headache or pain in your eye or eyebrow, nausea, blurred vision, or rainbow halos around lights. If you experience any of these, seek immediate medical care.

If you've received a diagnosis of glaucoma, establish a regular schedule of examinations with your doctor to be sure your treatment is helping maintain a safe pressure in your eyes.

Determining your risk

There's no specific test to prove you have glaucoma. A diagnosis is established by the amount of damage occurring to the optic nerve. When a doctor examines the retina, the optic disk will appear indented, or excavated, as if someone has scooped out part of its center. This sign is known as cupping (see photo on page 95), and results from the death of nerve cells. The normal contour and color

of the disk also may be affected by the loss of nerve fibers.

Two other factors also are often present and can help with a diagnosis:
- High intraocular pressure
- Areas of vision loss

Abnormally high IOP is frequently, but not always, associated with glaucoma. Generally, a perimetry test will reveal a loss of peripheral vision

Several tests, some done at a regular eye exam, can indicate risks of glaucoma by revealing elevated intraocular pressure, a thinning cornea or changes to the optic nerve:

Tonometry. Tonometry is a simple, painless procedure that measures your intraocular pressure. It's usually the initial screening test for glaucoma (see page 20). For the test, your doctor has you sit at a slit lamp, where a small flat-tipped cone pushes lightly against your eyeball. The force required to flatten (applanate) a small area of your cornea translates into a measure of your intraocular pressure.

A variety of other factors may cause tonometry readings to vary somewhat, including the thickness of your cornea and whether you previously had corneal laser surgery. For these reasons, newer technologies are being investigated to improve the standard applanation instrument and obtain more accurate measurements.

Visual field test. To check if glaucoma has affected your visual field, an exam using an automated perimeter is often performed (see page 15). You're seated in front of a lighted bowl on which bright points of light flash on and off. You'll be asked to press a button whenever you notice one of these flashes come into your visual field. Your responses are analyzed and compared to map your entire visual field.

Test for optic nerve damage. To check the fibers in your optic nerve, your doctor uses an instrument called an ophthalmoscope, or biomicroscope, which enables him or her to look directly through the pupil to the back of your eye. Your doctor may also use imaging techniques such as optical coherence tomography to create a three-dimensional image of your optic nerve. This image can reveal

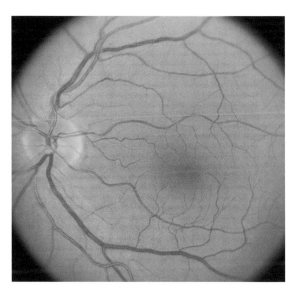 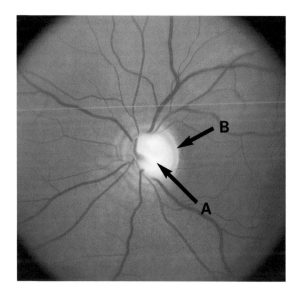

Optic nerve damage

The optic disk of a healthy eye (left) has an even reddish coloration. An optic disk affected by advanced glaucoma is excavated, or cupped, at the center of the disk (arrow A). Only a narrow rim of tissue remains on the optic nerve's edge (arrow B).

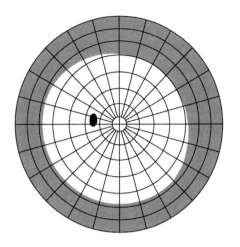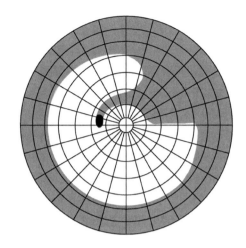

Visual field map

A normal visual field of the left eye mapped by tangent screen perimetry is shown at left (see page 15). The black spot near the center marks your normal blind spot — the location of the optic nerve. The visual field at right shows a typical pattern associated with glaucoma. Shading indicates that the upper right portion of the visual field has been lost.

slight changes to the fibers, indicating the earliest beginnings of glaucoma. Your doctor may take photographs of the optic nerve to be able to make comparisons at future visits and monitor any changes that could occur.

Pachymetry. The thickness of your cornea is an important factor for accurately diagnosing glaucoma — generally, the thinner the cornea, the greater your risk of having glaucoma. Your eye doctor may perform a test called pachymetry (puh-KIM-uh-tree)

that uses an ultrasound instrument to gauge the cornea's thickness. Keep in mind, thicker corneas may cause your eye pressure readings to seem high even though you don't have glaucoma. Conversely, thinner corneas may produce pressure readings that seem low but you may have glaucoma.

An additional test. Your doctor may use a technique called gonioscopy (go-nee-OS-kuh-pee), in which a special lens is placed on the eye to inspect the drainage angle.

Treatment

If your doctor determines that you have an excavated optic disk, you'll most likely be treated for glaucoma. If you have only slightly elevated IOP, an undamaged optic nerve and no visual field loss, you may not need treatment but more frequent eye examinations may be advised. If you have signs of optic nerve damage and visual field loss, even if your IOP is in the normal range, you may receive treatment to lower eye pressure further, which may help slow the progression of glaucoma.

Glaucoma can't be cured, and damage caused by the disease can't be reversed. But with treatment, glaucoma can be controlled. The way to preserve vision is by reducing intraocular pressure — either by improving the outflow of aqueous humor or by reducing the production of aqueous humor or both. Doctors may prescribe eyedrops, oral medications, laser treatment, incisional surgery or a combination of therapies.

When determining your treatment plan, factors often considered include your overall health, psychosocial issues and the risk of side effects. Because the disease can subtly progress or change, treatment may need adjustment over time. Regular checkups and adherence to a plan may seem burdensome, but they're essential to prevent vision loss.

Your eye doctor will likely begin treatment by identifying a baseline for your intraocular pressure. This may be obtained by measuring your IOP several times and at different times of the day.

Next, your doctor will establish a lower IOP that's unlikely to cause further damage to the optic nerve. This level is often referred to as the target pressure and may be a range rather than a single number. Target pressure differs depending on the amount of damage to your optic nerve and other factors. Your target pressure may change over the course of your lifetime.

Topical eye medications are the most common early treatment for glaucoma. Standard practice is to perform surgery only if these medications are ineffective or if the individual will have difficulty adhering to the recommended therapy. However, surgery can also be a relatively safe and effective initial treatment.

Eyedrops

Use of medicated eyedrops is often the first step in treatment for glaucoma. There are several types of drops that a doctor may prescribe (see pages 100-101). On occasions when a single medication isn't effective, a combination medication may be used.

It's important to use the drops exactly as prescribed to control your IOP. Skipping even a few doses can worsen the damage to your optic nerve. Some drops may need to be applied several times each day, while others are used just one time a day. Inform your doctor of other medications you're taking, to avoid any undesirable drug interactions.

Because some of the eyedrop fluid is absorbed into your bloodstream, you may experience certain side effects unrelated to your eyes. To minimize this absorption, close your eyes for a minute or two after putting the drops in. Press lightly at the corner of your eye near your nose to close the tear duct, and wipe off any unused drops from your eyelid.

Oral medications

If eyedrops alone don't bring your eye pressure down to the target level, your doctor may prescribe an oral medication. These medications are generally considered short-term therapy and prescribed as a transition stage to laser therapy or surgery.

The most common oral medications for glaucoma are from a class of drugs known as carbonic anhydrase inhibitors. They include acetazolamide and methazolamide. Take these pills with meals to reduce side effects. You can help to minimize the potassium loss that these medications can cause by adding bananas and apple juice to your diet.

When you first start taking oral medications, you may experience a frequent need to urinate and a tingling sensation in your fingers and toes. These symptoms will usually disappear after a few days. Other possible side effects from taking carbonic anhydrase inhibitors include rashes, depression, fatigue, lethargy, kidney stones, stomach upset, impotence, weight loss and a metallic taste in your mouth when drinking carbonated beverages.

Neuroprotective drugs

When it comes to preserving vision in people with glaucoma, lowering intraocular pressure provides only a partial solution. Another approach is treatment directed specifically at the optic nerve. Several clinical trials are under way to examine whether certain drugs may help protect the nerve fibers. One trial is investigating the potential neuroprotective effect of memantine (Namenda), an oral medication used in the treatment of Alzheimer's disease. Results from this study are still preliminary.

Laser therapy

In the last couple of decades, a procedure called trabeculoplasty (truh-BEK-u-lo-plas-tee) has been used to treat open-angle glaucoma. The doctor uses a high-energy laser beam to remodel and clear part of the trabecular meshwork. This helps aqueous humor drain more easily from the eye.

This form of laser therapy is generally an office procedure that takes 10 to 20 minutes. You'll likely be given an anesthetic eyedrop, seated at a slit lamp and fitted with a special lens on

Emergency care for glaucoma

Acute angle-closure glaucoma is a medical emergency. When you arrive at a hospital or clinic with this condition, doctors may administer several medications in an attempt to reduce your eye pressure as quickly as possible.

Once your eye pressure is under control, you may have an operation called an iridotomy (ir-ih-DOT-uh-mee). In this procedure, a laser beam creates a small hole in your iris to allow aqueous humor to flow more freely into the anterior chamber where it has normal access to the trabecular meshwork. If aqueous humor can reach the meshwork again, the fluid drains as it normally does. Many doctors recommend an iridotomy on the other eye at a later date because of the high risk that it too will undergo an attack within the next few years.

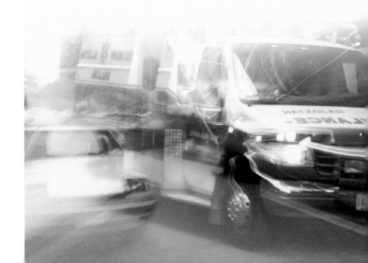

Eyedrops for glaucoma

Your doctor may prescribe more than one type of eyedrop. If you're using more than one, wait several minutes between applications of different eyedrops. The types of eyedrops that doctors most commonly prescribe include:

Name	Function	Drug names
Beta blockers	Reduce the production of aqueous humor	Betaxolol (Betoptic), carteolol (Ocupress), levobunolol (Betagan), metipranolol (OptiPranolol), timolol (Betimol, Timoptic)
Alpha-adrenergic agents	Reduce the production of aqueous humor	Apraclonidine (Iopidine), brimonidine (Alphagan P)
Carbonic anhydrase inhibitors	Reduce the amount of aqueous humor	Dorzolamide (Trusopt), brinzolamide (Azopt)
Prostaglandin analogues	Increase the outflow of aqueous humor	Latanoprost (Xalatan), bimatoprost (Lumigan), travoprost (Travatan)
Miotics (rarely used today)	Increase the outflow of aqueous humor	Pilocarpine (Isopto Carpine, Pilocar, others)
Epinephrine compounds (rarely used today)	Increase the outflow of aqueous humor	Epinephrine

Possible side effects

Difficulty breathing, slowed pulse, hair loss, decrease in blood pressure, impotence, fatigue, weakness, depression and memory loss. If you have asthma, bronchitis or emphysema, or if you have diabetes and use insulin, other medications may be recommended because beta blockers may worsen breathing problems.

Fatigue, dizziness, red, itchy or swollen eyes, dry mouth and allergic reactions.

Side effects are rare. If you're allergic or sensitive to sulfa drugs, this type of medication shouldn't be used unless there's no alternative, and then only with great care. (When a carbonic anhydrase inhibitor is taken orally, frequent urination and a tingling sensation in the fingers and the toes are common).

Mild reddening and stinging of the eyes and darkening of the iris, changes in the pigment of the eyelid skin, longer and thicker eyelashes, and blurred vision from swelling of the retina in rare cases.

Pain around or inside the eyes, brow ache, blurred or dim vision, nearsightedness, allergic reactions, stuffy nose, sweating, increased salivation and occasional digestive problems.

Red eyes, allergic reactions, heart palpitations, increase in blood pressure, headache and anxiety.

your eye. You'll see bright flashes of light as the doctor aims the laser through the lens and applies heat to the meshwork.

Often, you can resume normal activities immediately without discomfort. The doctor will likely check your eye pressure a couple of hours after the procedure and several times in the following weeks. It will take a few weeks before the full effect of the surgery becomes apparent.

If you have glaucoma in both eyes, the first eye will be treated and allowed to heal before the second eye is treated. Laser surgery for glaucoma usually lowers intraocular pressure initially. After a period of time, however, the pressure may gradually begin to increase.

Surgery

Surgery may be necessary to treat glaucoma if medications aren't effective or well tolerated. Surgery helps reduce the resistance to aqueous humor draining from the eye. Different procedures may be used. They may not eliminate the need for eyedrops or oral medications to maintain intraocular pressure.

Incisional surgery. An operation called a trabeculectomy (truh-bek-u-LEK-tuh-mee) may be used to help you control your eye pressure. This procedure may be done in a hospital or at an outpatient surgery center.

Beforehand, you'll likely receive a medication to help you relax. Your eye will be anesthetized with an injection. Using delicate instruments under an operating microscope, the surgeon creates a flap in the upper layer of the sclera — the white of your eye. Beneath the flap, the doctor removes a small piece of the sclera and trabecular meshwork, allowing aqueous humor to freely drain through this hole. The flap and the conjunctiva cover and protect the hole. This procedure works best if you haven't had any previous surgery on the eye.

Your doctor will likely check your eye in several follow-up visits. He or she will likely prescribe antibiotic and anti-inflammatory eyedrops to be used after the operation to help fight infection and prevent scarring of the newly created opening. Scarring is a particular problem for young adults, blacks and people who've had previous eye surgery.

Although incisional surgery may preserve existing vision, it can't restore vision that's already been lost. Sometimes, a single procedure may not lower eye pressure enough, in which case you may need to continue using glaucoma eyedrops or have another operation.

Drainage implants. With this procedure, the doctor inserts a small silicone tube in your eye to help drain aqueous humor. After the surgery you'll wear an eye patch for 24 hours and use eyedrops for several weeks to fight infection and scarring. Your doctor will check your eyes several times in the weeks that follow.

With any type of surgery, there's always a risk of complications. Possible complications from glaucoma surgery may include infection, bleeding, IOP that remains too high or too low, and possible loss of vision. Having eye surgery can also speed up the development of cataracts. Most of these complications can be effectively treated.

Newer types of surgery that pose fewer risks and allow for more consistent control of eye pressure are being investigated.

Prevention

Until recently, there was no proven way to prevent glaucoma. But one study found that cholesterol-lowering medications reduced the risk of open-angle glaucoma, especially among individuals who already have cardiovascular disease. This may be an added benefit for those already taking these medications, but more studies are needed to confirm the reduced risk and long-term efficacy.

Regular checkups also can help detect glaucoma in its early stages before irreversible vision loss has occurred. Follow the recommendations for checkups on pages 93-94.

Self-care

The most important thing that you can do if you have glaucoma is to keep yourself in good health and take your medications exactly as prescribed. Frequent eye exams will help your doctor monitor your eye pressure and keep you and your doctor aware of any changes to your vision. Other self-care tips include:

Maintain a healthy diet. Eat a diet full of fruits and vegetables to ensure that you're getting enough vitamins and minerals. Drink fluids in small amounts over the course of a day. Drinking a quart or more of any liquid within a short time may increase eye pressure. Limiting caffeine to low or moderate levels may be helpful.

Get regular exercise. People with open-angle glaucoma who exercise regularly — at least three times a week — may be able to moderately reduce their eye pressure. However, angle-closure glaucoma isn't affected by exercise, and people with pigmentary glaucoma, a form of secondary glaucoma, may experience increased eye pressure after exercise. In addition, yoga and other exercises that put you in a head-down position may increase the pressure in your eyes. Talk to your doctor about an appropriate exercise program.

Don't depend on herbal remedies. A number of herbal supplements, such as bilberry, are advertised as glaucoma remedies. Bilberry hasn't been proved effective at preventing or treating glaucoma and shouldn't be used in place of proven therapies. Be cautious about herbal supplements and discuss them with your doctor before trying them.

Find healthy ways to cope with stress. Stress can trigger an attack of acute angle-closure glaucoma. Relaxation techniques, such as meditation and progressive muscle relaxation, may help you deal with stress.

Wear proper eye protection. Eye trauma can cause an elevated IOP. Wear safety glasses or goggles when you play sports, use tools or machinery, or work with chemicals. When you're in the sun, even for only a few minutes, wear sunglasses that block ultraviolet (UV) light.

Chapter 6

Cataracts

A cataract is a clouding of the normally clear lens of the eye. The Latin word *cataracta* means "waterfall" — referring perhaps to the difficulty someone might have trying to see through a sheet of falling water. A better analogy might be trying to peer through a frosted or fogged-up window. Clouded vision makes it difficult to read, drive a car, do detail work or recognize a friend's face.

Clouding of the lens is normal as you get older. About half of Americans older than 65 have some degree of clouding of the lens. Most cataracts develop slowly and don't disturb your eyesight early on. After age 75, perhaps 70 percent of Americans have cataracts that are significant enough to impair their vision.

How you deal with cataracts is dependent on their severity and on your tolerance of blurred vision. In the early stages, cataracts are often left untreated as stronger lighting and eyeglasses can help you adjust to vision problems. But at some point — when your vision becomes moderately to significantly impaired and begins to jeopardize your normal lifestyle — you may need to seek treatment, which usually involves surgery. Fortunately, cataract removal is one of the safest, most effective and most common surgical procedures, restoring sight to millions of Americans.

Types of cataracts

A cataract can develop in one or both eyes, and it may or may not affect the entire lens. The eye's lens is located just behind the iris and the pupil. The lens is shaped much like a magnifying glass — it's thicker in the middle and thinner near the edges. Tiny ligaments, bands of tough fibrous tissue, hold the lens in place. When your eyes work properly, light passes through the cornea and the pupil to the lens. The lens focuses this light, producing clear, sharp images on the retina, the light-sensitive membrane on the inside of your eyeball that functions like the film of a camera.

When a cataract develops, the lens becomes clouded. The clouding scatters the light passing through it and prevents a sharply defined image from reaching the retina. The result is your vision becomes blurred. The greater the clouding, the greater the loss of vision.

Cataract myths

Perhaps because cataracts are one of the most common eye disorders, there are many misconceptions about them. Here are some of the facts:

- A cataract is not a film covering the outside of your eye. It's located within the eye — in the lens.
- Just because your eye looks clear doesn't mean there's no cataract. Most cataracts are detectable only with special instruments.
- Cataracts aren't caused by cancer.
- Cataracts don't spread from one eye to the other, although both eyes may be affected.
- Overusing your eyes doesn't cause cataracts.
- You don't have to wait for a cataract to turn completely white or become "ripe" before having it removed.

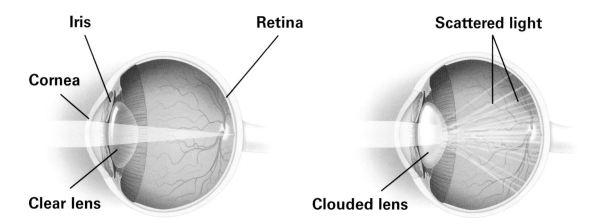

Iris Retina

Cornea

Clear lens

Scattered light

Clouded lens

How cataracts affect vision

A cataract occurs when the normally clear lens of your eye becomes cloudy. The clouding blurs vision by scattering the light passing through the lens — which prevents the lens from properly focusing an image on the retina.

The lens consists of three layers (see illustration on page 108). Accordingly, there are three types of cataracts, identified by the layer of the lens in which they develop. The outer layer is a thin membrane called the capsule. It surrounds a soft, clear material called the cortex. The hard center of the lens is the nucleus. If you think of the lens as a piece of fruit, the capsule is the skin, the cortex is the fleshy fruit, and the nucleus is the pit.

Each of these three types of cataracts can develop alone, or they can form in combination — more than one type can form in the lens at the same time.

Nuclear

A nuclear cataract, which occurs in the center of the lens, is the most common type of cataract and the one most associated with aging. Changes to the lens make the nucleus more compressed and less flexible. In the early stages, as the lens changes the way it focuses light, you may become more nearsighted or experience a temporary improvement in your reading vision. Some people actually stop needing their glasses. Unfortunately, this so-called second sight disappears as the normally clear lens gradually turns yellow or greenish and begins to cloud vision. As the cataract progresses, the lens may even turn brown. Seeing in dim light and driving at night can be difficult.

Cortical

A cortical cataract begins as whitish, wedge-shaped streaks on the outer edge of the cortex. As the condition progresses, the streaks extend to the center of the lens and interfere with light passing through the nucleus. Both your distance and near vision can be impaired. Focusing problems and distortion are common. You may also have problems with glare and loss of contrast. Many people with diabetes develop cortical cataracts. Cortical cataracts are the only type of cataract associated with exposure to ultraviolet (UV) light.

Subcapsular

A subcapsular cataract typically starts as a small, opaque area just under the capsular shell. It usually forms at the back of the lens, in the pathway of light headed to the retina. A subcapsular cataract may occur in both eyes but tends to be more advanced in one eye. It may interfere with reading, reduce vision in bright light, and pro-

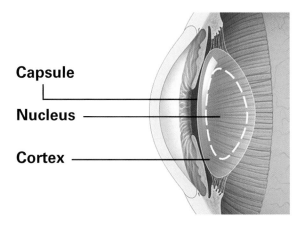

Capsule

Nucleus

Cortex

Parts of the lens

A cataract may develop as a normal part of aging. It can form in any one of the layers of the lens — the nucleus, the cortex or the capsule.

duce glare or halos around lights at night. You're more likely to develop a subcapsular cataract if you have diabetes, are very nearsighted, have taken corticosteroid drugs, or have had an eye injury or eye surgery.

Signs and symptoms

A cataract usually develops slowly and causes no pain. At first, the cloudiness may affect only a small

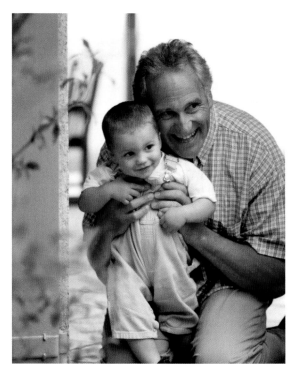 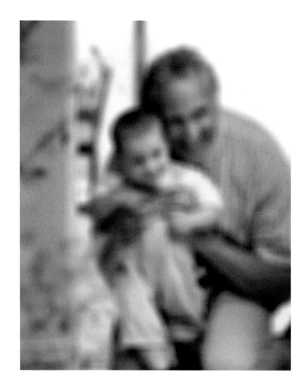

Vision with cataracts

A clouded lens from a cataract progressively turns clear normal vision (left) into blurred or dimmed vision (right).

part of the lens and you may be unaware of any changes in your vision. Over time, however, as the cataract grows and becomes larger, it affects more of the lens. When significantly less light is able to reach the retina, your vision becomes impaired.

The signs and symptoms of a cataract may include the following:

- Clouded, blurred or dim vision
- Increasing difficulty with night vision
- Sensitivity to light and glare
- Halos around lights
- Need for brighter light for reading and other activities
- Frequent changes in eyeglass or contact lens prescriptions
- Fading or yellowing of colors
- Double vision in one eye

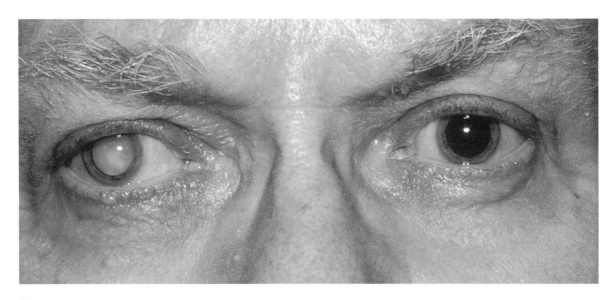

Hypermature cataract

An overripe (hypermature) cataract occurs when a lens becomes completely clouded, giving the pupil a white appearance. The condition should be treated quickly.

If you have a cataract, light from the sun, lamps or oncoming headlights may seem too bright. Glare and halos around lights can make driving uncomfortable and dangerous. You may experience eyestrain or find yourself blinking more often to clear your vision.

Signs and symptoms such as pain, redness, itching, irritation or a discharge from the eye aren't generally associated with a cataract but may be related to another eye disorder. A cataract isn't dangerous to the health of your eye unless it becomes completely white, known as an overripe (hypermature) cataract. This can cause inflammation, pain and headache. A hypermature cataract is extremely rare and should be removed as quickly as possible.

Causes

As you age, the lenses in your eyes become less flexible, less transparent and thicker. The lens is made mostly of water and protein fibers. The protein fibers are arranged in a precise manner that makes the lens clear and allows light to pass through without interference. With aging, the composition of the lens undergoes changes and the structure of the protein fibers breaks down. Some of the fibers begin to clump together, clouding small areas of the lens. As a cataract continues to develop, the clouding becomes more dense and involves a greater part of the lens.

Scientists don't know the reasons why a lens changes with age. One possibility could be from damage caused by unstable molecules known as free radicals. Smoking and exposure to UV light are two sources of free radicals. General wear and tear on the lens over the years also may cause changes in protein fibers.

You don't have to be an older adult to develop a cataract — they may start at an early age. But such cataracts tend to be small and develop slowly, so they often don't affect vision until after a person is age 60 or older. Some people are born with cataracts or develop them during childhood. Such cataracts may be the result of the mother having contracted rubella (German measles) during pregnancy. They may also be due to metabolic disorders. Congenital cataracts, as they're called, don't always affect vision, but if they do they're usually removed soon after detection.

Secondary cataracts can form as a complication of disease such as diabetes. They may also develop years after eye trauma and injury. Some types of radiation may cause cataracts.

Risk factors

Everyone is at risk of developing cataracts simply because age is the single greatest risk factor. By age 65 about half of all Americans have developed some degree of lens clouding, although it may not impair vision. Cataracts are slightly more common in women than in men, and they're more common in blacks than in whites.

Other factors that may increase your risk of cataracts include:
• Diabetes
• Family history of cataracts
• Previous eye surgery

- Previous eye injury or inflammation
- Prolonged use of corticosteroids
- Excessive exposure to sunlight
- Smoking
- Excessive consumption of alcohol

Screening and diagnosis

The only way to know for certain if you have a cataract is to have an eye examination that includes a visual acuity test, a slit-lamp examination and a retinal examination (see pages 16-19). During an eye exam, your pupil generally is dilated to examine the lens for signs of a cataract and, if needed, determine how dense the clouding is. Your eye doctor likely will also check for glaucoma and, if you have blurred vision or discomfort, for other problems with the retina and the optic nerve.

If you have a cataract, you can discuss treatment options with your eye doctor. If, in addition to having a cataract, you have another serious eye condition, removing the cataract may not result in improved vision.

Treatment

The only effective treatment for a cataract is surgery to remove the clouded lens and replace it with a clear lens implant. Cataracts can't be cured with medications, dietary supplements, exercise or optical devices.

In the early stages of a cataract when symptoms are mild, a good understanding of the condition and a willingness to adjust your lifestyle can help. Here are a few simple steps for dealing with the symptoms:

- If you have eyeglasses or contact lenses, make sure they're the most accurate prescription possible.
- Use a magnifying glass to read.
- Improve the lighting in your home with more or brighter lamps, for example, ones that can accommodate halogen lights or 100- to 150-watt incandescent bulbs.
- When you go outside during the day, wear sunglasses to reduce glare.
- Limit your night driving.

These measures may help for a while, but as the cataract progresses, your vision will likely deteriorate further.

When vision loss starts to interfere with your daily activities, you'll want to consider cataract surgery. More than 1.5 million cataract surgeries are performed each year. Surgery is very successful in restoring vision.

More than 95 percent of people who have a cataract removed enjoy improved vision. In addition to better vision, many people find they need less powerful eyeglass prescriptions and have an improved quality of life.

An eye on history

Years ago, having a cataract removed was an ordeal involving several days in the hospital, painful stitches in the eye and a recovery spent lying on your back with your head held in place with sandbags. Luckily, the procedure has changed dramatically.

Modern surgical treatment of cataracts started with the development of the intraocular lens in 1949 by Harold Ridley, M.D., an English ophthalmologist. Dr. Ridley recalled the experiences of eye doctors who had treated Royal Air Force pilots during World War II. Some pilots had bits of hard plastic lodged in their eye after their plane's cockpit shattered. To the doctors' surprise, these fragments didn't cause any serious problems in the pilots' eyes. With this in mind, Dr. Ridley began experimenting with making artificial lenses from plastic.

In the mid-1960s American ophthalmologist Charles Kelman, M.D., developed phacoemulsification, a surgical procedure in which the cataract is removed while leaving the capsule surrounding the lens in place. Since then, advances in surgical techniques and lens replacement have made cataract surgery one of the safest and most effective surgeries. The number of cataract surgeries done each year has increased phenomenally in the United States and Europe.

And what does the future hold? One area of research is the use of lasers in phacoemulsification. Other surgical techniques are being investigated, and researchers are also looking at ways to prevent cataract formation with drugs.

Choosing the right time for surgery

The decision to have cataract surgery is one that you and your eye doctor make together. You'll probably have plenty of time to consider and discuss your options carefully — there should be no rush. In most cases, waiting until you're ready to have surgery won't harm your eye. You may not need cataract surgery for many years, if at all. In younger people or people with diabetes, however, cataracts may develop earlier and more quickly.

Base the decision on your degree of vision loss and your ability to function in daily life. Think about how the cataract affects what you do routinely. Can you see to perform your job or drive safely? Do you have problems reading or watching television? Is it difficult to cook, shop, do yardwork, climb stairs or take medications? How active are you, and does lack of vision affect your level of independence? Are you afraid you'll trip or fall or bump into something?

The answers to these questions are different for each person. A retired person who is no longer very active may have less need for sharp vision than does a younger person who needs to drive a car and earn a living. Some people with only minor vision loss from a cataract might want surgery because of problems with glare or double vision. Sometimes, a cataract should be removed even if it doesn't cause major problems with vision — for example, if it's interfering with the treatment of another eye problem, such as age-related macular degeneration, diabetic retinopathy or retinal detachment.

If you have cataracts in both eyes and decide to have surgery, your eye doctor typically removes the cataract in one eye at a time. This allows time for the first eye to heal before the second eye surgery takes place.

The surgical procedure

Two things happen during cataract surgery — the clouded lens is removed, and an artificial lens is implanted. Advances in surgical technique and more sophisticated technology have helped make this surgery a safe and effective procedure.

Before performing the surgery, your eye doctor measures the size and

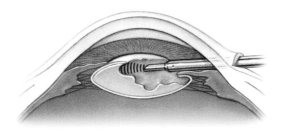

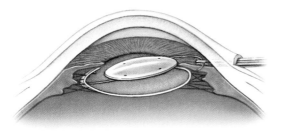

Phacoemulsification

During the phacoemulsification procedure, the rapidly vibrating tip of an ultrasound probe breaks up the cataract, which the surgeon then suctions out (top). After removing the clouded lens, your surgeon delicately inserts a lens implant into the empty capsule that still remains following the procedure (bottom).

shape of your eye to determine the correct power for the lens implant. This measurement is made with a painless ultrasound test. Cataract surgery is typically an outpatient procedure that takes less than an hour. Most people are relaxed and comfortable during the surgery, needing only local anesthesia. On rare occasions,

some people may need to be put under general anesthesia.

There are different types of surgical procedures that may be used to remove a cataract.

Phacoemulsification. The most commonly used form of cataract surgery is phacoemulsification (fak-o-e-mul-sih-fih-KA-shun). During this procedure, the surgeon breaks up and removes the cataract while leaving most of the outer layer (lens capsule) in place. The capsule helps support the lens implant when it's inserted.

The surgeon makes a small incision, about 1/8 inch (3 mm), where the cornea meets the conjunctiva and inserts a needle-thin probe. The surgeon then uses the probe, which vibrates with ultrasound waves, to break up (emulsify) the cataract and suction out the fragments.

Extracapsular cataract extraction. If your cataract has advanced beyond the point where phacoemulsification can effectively break up the clouded lens, the surgeon may do an extracapsular cataract extraction. This procedure requires a larger incision, about 3/8 inch (10 mm), where the cornea and sclera meet. Through this incision the surgeon opens the lens capsule, removes the nucleus in one piece and vacuums out the lens cortex, leaving the capsule shell in place.

Once the cataract has been removed through the phacoemulsification or extracapsular method, a clear artificial lens is implanted into the empty lens capsule to replace the original

New options with intraocular lenses

Most lens implants, or intraocular lenses (IOLs), are monofocal, that is, they have a fixed point of focus for either near vision or distance vision. If a distance lens is implanted, you'll need to wear glasses or contact lenses for reading; if a reading lens is implanted, you'll need glasses for driving. Most of the monofocal lenses that are implanted for cataracts correct for distance vision.

A variety of lens implants, called multifocal IOLs, have been developed that give you much greater flexibility and convenience. One type of lens is made with zones of different refractive power, much like the progressive lenses used in eyeglasses. Another type of

multifocal IOL is the accommodative lens that shifts in the eye to change the refractive power. This shift is in response to movements of the eye's ciliary muscles, mimicking the eye's natural accommodative abilities. Recently, the Food and Drug Administration (FDA) approved products of both multifocal types.

The primary goal of the multifocal IOL is to provide you with good visual acuity at more than one distance without the aid of eyeglasses and contact lenses. Clinical trials demonstrated that most recipients of an accommodating lens had improved vision at faraway, intermediate and close distances.

clouded lens. This lens implant, known as an intraocular lens (IOL), is made of plastic, acrylic or silicone. It requires no care and becomes a permanent part of your eye.

Some IOLs are rigid plastic and implanted through an incision that requires several stitches (sutures) to close. However, many IOLs are flexible, allowing a smaller incision that

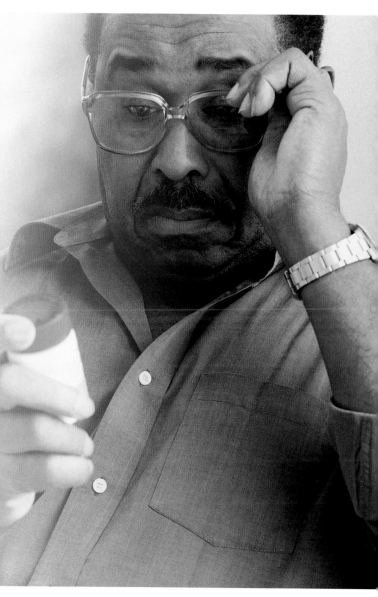

However, you can never be 100 percent certain of seeing well without eyeglasses or contact lenses after cataract surgery. For example, your distance vision may improve but perhaps not as much as if you would have a monofocal IOL corrected for distance. Some people with multifocal IOLs experience problems with glare, night driving, halos around lights and loss of contrast.

Other advances in intraocular lenses include development of toric IOLs to correct astigmatism. As surgical techniques continue to improve, foldable intraocular lenses are being used that can be placed through even smaller incisions.

requires no stitches. The surgeon can fold this type of lens and insert it into the empty capsule where the natural lens used to be. Once in place, the lens unfolds.

After cataract surgery

With phacoemulsification and foldable lens implants, surgical incisions have become very small and often no sutures are required. If all goes well, you'll heal fast and your vision will start to improve after several days. If your surgery requires a larger incision and sutures, full healing might take a little longer.

Normally you can go home on the same day as surgery, but you won't

Second cataract

What's a second cataract, or "aftercataract?" This condition occurs when the back of the lens capsule — the part of the lens that isn't removed during surgery and that supports the lens implant — eventually becomes cloudy and blurs your vision. Another term for this condition is posterior capsule opacification (PCO). This opacification can develop months or years after cataract surgery. It happens about 25 percent of the time. The gradual clouding is the result of cell growth on the back of the lens capsule.

Treatment for PCO is simple and quick. It involves a technique called YAG laser capsulotomy, in which a laser beam makes a small opening in the clouded capsule to let light pass through. *Capsulotomy* means "cutting into the capsule," and YAG is an acronym for yttrium, aluminum and garnet, the laser used for this procedure.

Laser capsulotomy is a quick, painless outpatient procedure. Afterward, you typically stay in the doctor's office for about an hour to make sure your eye pressure isn't elevated. In some people, particularly those who have glaucoma or are extremely nearsighted, YAG laser surgery can raise eye pressure. Other complications are rare but can include swelling of the macula and a detached retina.

be able to drive, so make sure to arrange for a ride home. You'll typically see your eye doctor the next day, the following week, and then again after a month so that he or she can check the healing progress.

It's normal to feel mild discomfort for a couple of days after surgery. Avoid rubbing or pressing on your eye. Clean your eyelids with soft tissue or cotton balls to remove any crusty discharge. You may wear an eye patch or protective shield the day of surgery. Your doctor may prescribe medications to prevent infection and control eye pressure. After a couple of days, all discomfort should diminish and disappear.

Contact your doctor immediately if you experience any of the following signs or symptoms after cataract surgery:
- Vision loss
- Pain that persists despite the use of over-the-counter pain medications
- A significant increase in eye redness
- Light flashes or multiple spots (floaters) in front of your eye
- Nausea, vomiting or excessive coughing

Most people need to wear eyeglasses after cataract surgery, no matter whether they wore glasses before. Astigmatism — a focusing problem that occurs when your cornea isn't curved evenly in all directions — is common after cataract surgery but less of a problem when the surgery involves a small incision. Your doctor will let you know when your eyes have healed enough for you to get a prescription for eyeglasses.

Complications after cataract surgery are relatively rare, and most can be treated. They include inflammation, infection, bleeding and swelling. The risks are greater for people who have other eye diseases or serious medical problems. Occasionally, cataract surgery fails to improve vision because of pre-existing conditions such as glaucoma or macular degeneration. It may be necessary to treat these other eye problems before proceeding with cataract surgery.

Prevention

Most cataracts occur with age and can't altogether be avoided. Regular eye exams remain the key to early detection. You can also take steps to help slow or prevent the development of a cataract:

- Don't smoke. Smoking produces the unstable molecules known as free radicals, increasing your risk of cataracts.
- Eat a balanced diet. Your daily diet should include plenty of fruits and vegetables.
- Use sun protection. Ultraviolet light may contribute to the development of cataracts. Whenever possible, wear sunglasses when you're outdoors.
- Take care of other health problems. Follow your treatment plan if you have diabetes or other medical conditions.

Researchers continue to explore new ways to prevent and treat cataracts, such as developing medications that would reduce or eliminate the need for surgery. But until such a medication exists, your chances of fully restoring your vision with cataract surgery are excellent if you have no other eye diseases.

Chapter 7

Protecting your sight

It's easy to take your vision for granted — until something happens that limits or impairs your ability to see clearly. Of course, everyone's vision changes with age, and not every eye problem or injury can be avoided. But good eye care goes a long way toward protecting your sight and reducing your risk of some eye diseases.

What is good eye care? It means having your vision checked regularly and keeping chronic medical conditions that can affect eyesight, such as diabetes and high blood pressure, under the best possible control. It means wearing protective eyewear in situations that may endanger your eyes. It means developing good work habits to avoid eyestrain. And it also means recognizing symptoms that may require immediate attention.

When it comes to your vision, it's "Better safe than sorry." It's far better to take the time and effort to do the little things that prevent eye injuries and problems than to adapt to life with vision impairment.

Get regular eye exams

An eye examination is one of the best ways to protect your vision. That's because it's so important to detect eye problems at the earliest stage — when they're usually most treatable. Chronic eye disorders such as macular degeneration, glaucoma and diabetic retinopathy can do serious, irreparable damage to your vision before you're aware of any symptoms. If you wait for symptoms to develop before seeing an eye doctor, you may have waited too long. Regular eye exams help:

- Detect problems at their earliest stages
- Correct vision changes brought on by aging
- Identify and reduce sources of eyestrain and fatigue
- Assure you that your vision is the best it can be

Who gives eye exams?

Routine eye care may involve three kinds of eye specialists: ophthalmologists, optometrists and opticians.

Ophthalmologists. Ophthalmologists are medical doctors with a thorough understanding of all serious eye conditions and the treatment options available. Ophthalmologists provide complete eye care. They can give you an eye exam and other vision services, prescribe corrective lenses, diagnose and treat complex eye disorders and perform surgery. Some ophthalmologists may limit the range of their services, for example treating only specific eye diseases or performing only a specific type of surgery.

Extensive training is required to become an ophthalmologist. After college, ophthalmologists must complete medical school, an internship and a residency program. In addition, some ophthalmologists choose to specialize in a specific area of care and treatment, which often requires additional training.

Optometrists. Optometrists are trained and licensed to provide many eye care services, such as evaluating your vision, prescribing corrective lenses, diagnosing common eye disorders and treating certain eye diseases with medications. For more complex eye problems or for conditions requiring surgery, you'll likely be referred to an ophthalmologist.

Opticians. Opticians fill prescriptions for eyeglasses and contact lenses — designing, finishing, fitting and dispensing. They assist optometrists and ophthalmologists in providing full vision services.

Ophthalmologists, optometrists and opticians generally work collaboratively with you to provide the best possible eye care. Consider their qualifications, experience and the services provided when selecting an individual or group practice for your eye care.

When to have an eye exam

How frequently you need an eye exam depends on several factors, including your age, health and risk of developing eye problems. The American Academy of Ophthalmology makes the following recommendations:

Children and adolescents. Young children should be screened for childhood eye disorders such as crossed eyes (strabismus), lazy eye

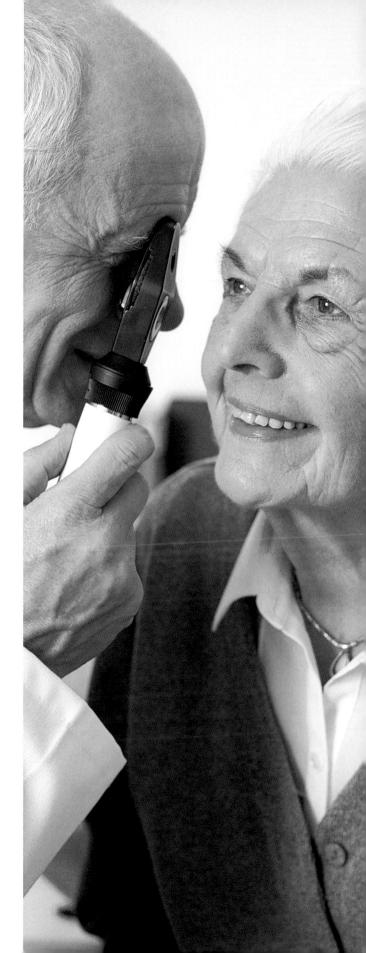

Signs of an eye emergency

If you notice any of these signs and symptoms, schedule an appointment with your eye doctor as soon as possible, even if you've recently had an eye exam:

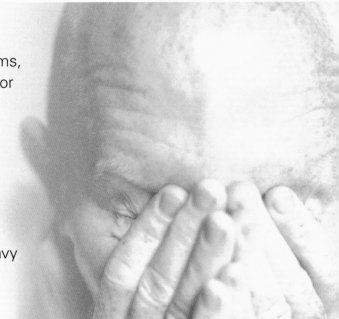

- Sudden onset of hazy or blurred vision
- Eye pain
- Flashes of light, dark spots or ghost-like images in your visual field
- Halos or rainbows form around lights
- Lines and edges appear distorted and wavy

Communicating with your eye doctor

Good communication between you and your doctor is essential for keeping your eyes healthy. Be prepared to discuss the following topics at an eye exam, particularly if it's been several years since your previous visit:

- Vision problems that you're currently having or have had in the recent past
- Satisfaction with your eyeglasses or contact lenses, if you wear them
- Health problems that you've had in recent years
- Medications you're currently taking
- Any allergies you may have to medication, food or other substances
- Family history of eye disease, such as cataracts or glaucoma
- Family history of systemic diseases that affect vision, such as diabetes, high blood pressure and heart disease

If you wear eyeglasses or contact lenses, bring them to your appointment. Your doctor will want to check them to make sure your prescription is the best one for you.

(amblyopia) and drooping eyelid (ptosis). They should also be tested for refractive errors such as nearsightedness, farsightedness and astigmatism. Eye exams should be scheduled:
- Between birth and 3 months
- Between 6 months and 1 year
- At about 3 years
- At about 5 years

Children between ages 6 and 19 should have their vision checked during regular medical appointments or if they experience blurred vision, eye pain, light flashes or excessive tearing. Exams are recommended for anyone with a disease that's known to put eyes at risk, such as diabetes.

Adults. If you experience no symptoms of vision loss and are at a low risk of eye disease, schedule an eye exam at the following intervals:
- At least once between ages 20 and 29
- At least twice between ages 30 and 39
- Every two to four years between ages 40 and 65
- Every one to two years over the age of 65

You may need more frequent eye exams if you have these risk factors:

- Personal or family history of eye disease
- Previous eye injury
- Systemic disease such as diabetes, high blood pressure, heart disease or acquired immunodeficiency syndrome (AIDS)
- You were born premature
- You're black and over age 40 (which puts you at high risk of glaucoma)

At the end of the eye exam, your doctor likely will provide you with a detailed assessment of your vision, along with any risks you should be concerned about and steps that you can take to protect your eyesight.

If your doctor gives you a prescription for corrective lenses, that doesn't automatically mean that you have to buy and use eyeglasses or contact lenses. If you have mild vision problems and your uncorrected vision isn't bothering you — you can still pass your driver's test and safely perform daily activities — you may not need to use corrective lenses. Going without them won't make your vision any worse. So don't let fears of being "trapped" into something you don't want to do prevent you from getting regular eye exams.

Use protective eyewear

One of the most effective ways to protect your vision is to wear safety glasses or goggles in situations that could potentially injure your eyes. According to the National Society to Prevent Blindness, the use of proper eye protection could have prevented nearly 90 percent of all impact injuries to the eye. Many of these injuries happen on the job or while participating in sports and recreational activities. Because extended exposure to sunlight can damage eyes, sunglasses also offer important protection.

At work

Power tools, heavy machinery, potent chemicals, flying particles of metal, glass and wood — these are among the workplace hazards that put your eyes at risk. According to the American Academy of Ophthalmology, each day more than 2,000 American workers injure their eyes in job-related accidents. Many workers had been using inappropriate eyewear or not wearing eye protection at all.

If your job carries a risk of eye injury, your employer is required by law to provide you with safety glasses. Workers in industrial settings, including anyone working with power tools, are required to wear them. A welder should wear a face shield to filter out the bright ultraviolet light of a welding arc. Eye protection is also important on farms and in shops or laboratories when you work with fertilizers, pesticides, caustic chemicals and solvents.

At home

Some of the most common eye injuries occur while people are performing everyday tasks at home. Spattered cooking grease, splashed detergent or drain cleaner, and sprayed garden chemicals are very harmful to eyes. So are disinfectants, solvents, oven cleaners, bleach and many other household products. Materials containing ammonia, chlorine, alkali or lye are especially dangerous. When you're using these products, protect yourself by wearing safety glasses or goggles, and if a child is helping you, make sure he or she wears protective eyewear as well. Remember to never mix cleaning agents together.

How to handle an eye injury

If an eye injury occurs, see an eye specialist immediately or go to an urgent care center or hospital emergency room. The full extent of the damage isn't always apparent — even what appears to be a minor injury may cause permanent damage if it's not treated.

If you sustain a blunt injury or cut to your eye:
- Cover the eye with some type of shield. For example, tape the bottom of a plastic or foam cup against your eye socket.
- Don't put any ointment or medication in the eye. Don't try to rinse the eye.
- Don't rub the eye. This could tear the tissue, causing more damage.
- Avoid taking aspirin, ibuprofen (Advil, Motrin, others) or other nonsteroidal anti-inflammatory drugs (NSAIDs). These medications thin the blood and may increase bleeding.

If you get a chemical in your eye:
- Rinse the eye with water to dilute and remove any chemical residue. Try to pull your eyelids open as wide as possible and flood the eye with a steady stream of water for at least 15 minutes. Tilt your head toward the injured side so that the chemical does not wash into the uninjured eye.
- After rinsing the eye, cover it with a soft pad. Take the chemical container with you to the emergency room, or write the product name on a slip of paper and take that.

If you have a foreign object in your eye:
- Don't try to remove anything that's on the cornea or that seems to be stuck or embedded in the white of the eye. Don't rub the eye. Cover both eyes with a soft pad.
- If the foreign object is floating on the white of the eye or inside the eyelid, try to remove it with the corner of a clean cloth, a tissue or a cotton swab.

It's always a good idea to wear protective eyewear for home repairs and hobbies. Whether you're repairing the car, painting the house or cleaning the garage, wear safety goggles to keep dirt, rust, paint chips and other small particles from landing in your eyes.

At play

Participation in sports and recreational activities can leave you with more than sore muscles or bruises. A ball, paintball or puck hitting your eye at high speed can cause serious damage. Finger pokes may scrape or tear your cornea. Water sports may lead to eye irritation or infection. According to the American Academy of Ophthalmology, each year more than 40,000 people experience sports-related eye injuries. Most injuries could have been prevented with impact-resistant eyewear made of polycarbonate plastic — regular eyeglasses and contact lenses don't provide enough protection.

Hard workouts may cause eyewear to fog up. If this happens, don't remove your eyewear for any reason during play. Wait until there's a break in the action or you have a chance to leave the game.

In the sun

Ultraviolet (UV) rays from the sun can damage your eyes as well as your skin. Artificial light sources such as welding arcs or tanning lamps are capable of burning the cornea and conjunctiva of your eye much like sunlight can. Long-term exposure to UV radiation increases your risk of eye disease, particularly cataracts and age-related macular degeneration.

The best way to protect your eyes from the sun is to wear sunglasses designed to block UV radiation and eliminate glare. The sunglasses don't have to be expensive to be effective. Look for ones that block 99 percent to 100 percent of both ultraviolet A (UVA) and ultraviolet B (UVB) light. To be even more effective, they should fit close to your face or have wraparound frames.

Wear sunglasses anytime you're outdoors for more than a few minutes. Remember to wear them even on cloudy days because clouds don't block all UV radiation.

You may reduce glare — the light that bounces off smooth surfaces such as pavement, water, sand and snow

— by choosing darker lenses that block more visible light. Polarized lenses also reduce reflected glare. But polarization doesn't block UV radiation, so if you're buying polarizing lenses, check the label to make sure that they also provide maximum UV protection.

Safe fun in the sun

Besides wearing sunglasses, follow these tips to keep your eyes protected from the sun:

- Wear a wide-brimmed hat or cap. Fifty percent of sunlight comes from directly overhead and can slip past most sunglasses.
- Never look at the sun directly, even through sunglasses, because doing so can permanently damage your eyes. You can also hurt your eyes by routinely staring at the sun reflected on water.
- Wear sunscreen on your face and around your eyes, including your eyelids.
- Avoid commercial tanning booths. If you do go, make sure the salon gives you special protective goggles to wear.
- Certain drugs make your eyes more sensitive to light. These photosensitizing drugs include tetracycline (Sumycin), doxycycline (Doryx, Monodox, Vibramycin) and phenothiazine derivatives, such as chlorpromazine (Thorazine) and thioridazine (Mellaril). Wear sunglasses and a hat each time you go outside for as long as you are taking one of these drugs.
- If you have an eye disease such as macular degeneration, you're at greater risk of UV-related eye damage. Protect your eyes whenever you go outside, no matter how briefly.

Avoiding eyestrain

Reading in dim light ruins your eyes, right? Wrong. That's a myth — the same as the belief that sitting too close to the TV screen or reading by flashlight harms your vision. These habits, while not advisable, won't permanently damage your eyes. However, any type of work that involves intensive use of your eyes, like reading, working at the computer or doing crafts, may cause eyestrain. Common signs and symptoms include:

- Sore, tired, burning or itching eyes
- Dry or watery eyes
- Blurred or double vision
- Headache and sore neck
- Difficulty shifting your focus
- Increased sensitivity to light

Shed light on the subject

When doing close-up work, make sure that you have light that's well directed on what you're doing. And, depending on your needs, don't be shy about increasing the wattage. Although a 60-watt to 100-watt light bulb may be sufficient for a person with normal vision, a 150-watt or 200-watt bulb may be necessary if you have reduced vision from conditions such as macular degeneration. Whenever you change a bulb, make sure the light fixture can handle the wattage of the new bulb.

When reading. When sitting, try to position the light source behind you and direct the light onto your page. The light should be bright but not glaring. If you're reading at a desk, use a shaded light positioned in front of you. The shade will keep light from shining directly into your eyes.

At the computer. Place your monitor so that the brightest light source is to the side. Check that the surrounding light is darker than the lightest part of your screen. Position adjustable lighting so that it doesn't shine into your eyes or reflect off the screen.

When watching television. Keep the room softly illuminated when you're watching TV. Too great a contrast between the screen and its surroundings can result in eyestrain.

Combat computer eyestrain

If you're seated in front of a computer monitor all day, you may experience the symptoms of eyestrain. You may have difficulty shifting your focus between the monitor and the documents on your desk. You may see color fringes or afterimages as you glance away from the monitor. Although the eyestrain isn't thought to have long-term consequences, the symptoms are unpleasant and disruptive. You may not be able to change the nature of your job, but you can take steps to reduce the strain.

Take eye breaks. Give your eyes a break by forcing them to focus on something other than your computer screen. Look away from the screen and at an object several feet away for 10 seconds every 10 minutes. Or look up from what you're doing and simply let your eyes unfocus.

Change the pace. Try to stand up and move around at least once every hour or so. If possible, lean back and close your eyes for a few moments. Give yourself a five-minute break every hour to do other work, such as phone calls and filing.

Blink often. Many people blink less than normal when working at the computer, which can result in dry, irritated eyes. Make a conscious effort

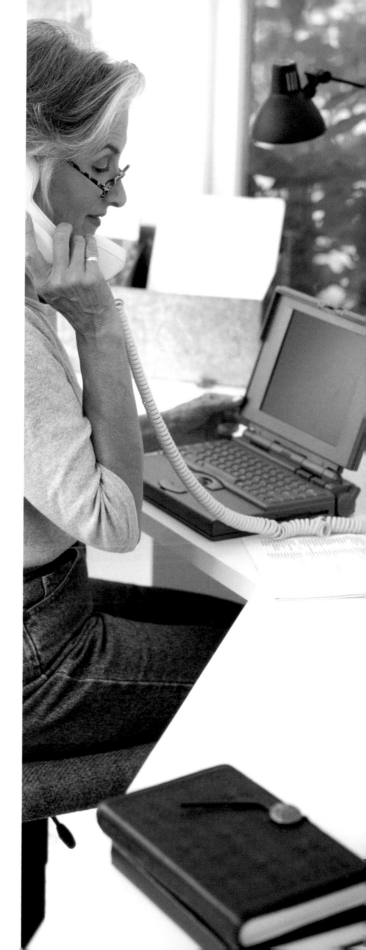

to blink more often to produce tears that can help moisten and lubricate your eyes. Consider regularly using artificial teardrops when you work at a computer for prolonged periods of time with few breaks.

Get appropriate eyewear. If you wear glasses or contacts, make sure the correction is right for computer work. Many lenses are intended for reading print close up, and they may not be optimal for hours spent on the computer.

Adjust your monitor. Position the monitor directly in front of you — about 20 to 28 inches from your eyes. Many people find that putting the screen at arm's length is about right. If you need to lean forward to read small type, consider increasing the font size or the page view.

The top of your screen should be at eye level or below so that you look down slightly at your work. If the monitor is too high or too low, it can lead to a sore neck.

Position your keyboard properly. Place the keyboard directly in front of your monitor. If the keyboard is at an angle or to the side, your eyes may

tire from having to constantly shift their focus.

Position reference materials nearby. Place books and papers on a document holder beside your monitor and at the same level, angle and distance from your eyes as the monitor. This way your eyes aren't constantly re-adjusting.

Reduce glare. Sit at your computer with the monitor off and note any areas of reflected light on the blank screen. These are the areas where glare can interfere with your ability to see clearly the words and images on your screen. The worst problems with glare are generally from sources above or behind you, including fluorescent lighting and sunlight.

Consider turning off some or all overhead lights. Close blinds and shades and avoid placing your monitor directly in front of a window or white wall. Use a glare-reducing screen and adjust the contrast or brightness of the monitor to a level that makes letters easy to read.

Wipe the dust from your screen regularly. Dust cuts down on contrast and may intensify glare on the screen.

Be careful with eyedrops

Mild eye discomfort, whether from eyestrain, dry eye, allergies or other causes, can be soothed with eyedrops. Three types of eyedrops are available without a prescription:

Decongestive eyedrops. Decongestive eyedrops, also called vasoconstrictors, whiten your eyes by shrinking the tiny blood vessels in the conjunctiva. One or two drops in your eye can relieve redness for several hours and often soothe irritation. Improvement should be prompt — and if not, check with an eye doctor to see whether this signals a more serious concern.

Allergy eyedrops. Some decongestive eyedrops include an antihistamine that provides added relief from seasonal allergies such as hay fever. Look for the word *allergy* on the label. Use allergy eyedrops no more than two or three times a day, unless instructed otherwise by your doctor.

Lubricating eyedrops. Lubricating eyedrops, also called artificial tears,

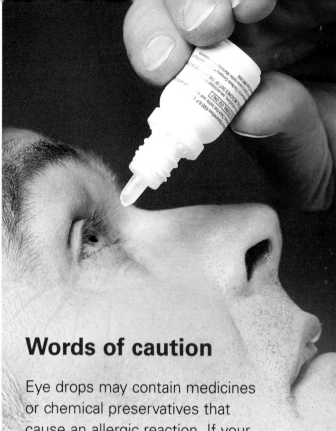

Words of caution

Eye drops may contain medicines or chemical preservatives that cause an allergic reaction. If your eyes or eyelids become more red, itchy or swollen after you apply eyedrops, stop using the drops and talk to your eye doctor.

Follow the recommended dosage for eyedrops. Using some drops more frequently can lead to problems. For example, if you use decongestive eyedrops too often, a rebound effect may occur — the redness and irritation increases after the drops wear off.

If you're at risk of angle-closure glaucoma, don't use eyedrops that contain antihistamines. They can provoke a glaucoma attack.

contain substances that help retain water and prevent it from evaporating, much as your own tears do. One or two drops of artificial tears can soothe irritated eyes, providing lubrication and comfort. You may apply these drops as often as needed.

How to use eyedrops

To administer eyedrops, follow these steps:

- Tilt your head back and gently pull your lower lid away from the eye to form a small pocket. Let the drop fall into the pocket. Don't let the tip of the bottle brush against your eye or eyelid.
- Close your eyes gently and don't blink. Don't squeeze the lids tightly shut, which may force some of the drop out of the eye.
- Use your index finger to apply pressure at the point where the lids meet the nose. This prevents the drop from draining immediately through the tear duct.
- Keep your eyes closed for a minute or two. Wipe any excess drops and tears from the closed lids with a tissue. Then open your eyes.

Eat a balanced diet

Hardly a week goes by without a new study touting the health benefits of various foods. So is there a healthy diet for your eyes? Scientists believe that one of the reasons why the mac-

Smoking and eye health

No discussion of good eye care would be complete without mentioning the hazards of smoking. Smoke, like any air pollutant, can irritate and redden your eyes as well as the eyes of people close by. What's more, smoking is a risk factor for cataracts, age-related macular degeneration, diabetic retinopathy, ischemic optic neuropathy and retinal vascular occlusions. Need another good reason to stop smoking? How about protecting your eyesight.

ula and other parts of the eye deterio-rate from the wear and tear of aging may stem from a lack of certain nutri-ents, including vitamins, carotenoids and minerals. Carotenoids (kuh-ROT-uh-noidz) aren't vitamins, but the body converts some of them into vita-mins, for example, turning beta carotene into vitamin A. These nutri-ents are highly concentrated in the retina and often fall to significantly lower levels when the macula starts to deteriorate.

Many carotenoids have antioxidant properties that help keep your body's cells healthy. Your body — and your eyes — use the antioxidants to com-bat unstable oxygen molecules in the bloodstream, called free radicals. Generally, free radicals perform a number of useful functions but a sur-plus can damage normal cells in a process called oxidation. Oxidation is thought to play a role in the develop-ment of macular degeneration, glau-coma and cataracts, as well as other conditions such as cardiovascular dis-ease and cancer.

For good eye health, try eating at least five servings of fruits and veg-etables each day. The wider the vari-ety of fruits and vegetables you

choose from, the better. The most col-orful fruits and vegetables — yellow, orange, red and dark green — con-tain nutrients that are the most highly concentrated in your eyes. This does-n't mean that they're the only ones you should eat. Most fresh produce is beneficial to your health.

What about nutritional supplements? Are they as good at preventing or stopping age-related eye disease as fresh produce? In general, supple-ments should be used to enhance nutrition but not replace real food. If you take a daily vitamin and mineral supplement, it's best not to exceed 100 percent of the Daily Value (DV) for each vitamin and mineral, unless your doctor advises otherwise. However, there's growing evidence that certain supplements, formulated in high-dose combinations, may be effective treatment options for certain eye conditions.

High-dose antioxidant combinations

Results from a study called the Age-Related Eye Disease Study (AREDS), funded by the National Eye Institute, provided encouraging news about protecting your vision with your diet.

The study involved individuals with dry macular degeneration, at different stages of the disease. Some participants were given a daily high-dose vitamin and mineral supplement that contained vitamin A (beta carotene), vitamin C, vitamin E, zinc and copper. Others were given an inactive pill (placebo). Over a five-year period, the participants were closely monitored, and outcomes from the two groups compared. Individuals taking the vitamin and mineral supplement were able to lower their risk of developing the advanced stages of macular degeneration by about 25 percent. People who took the supplement also reduced their risk of vision loss due to macular degeneration by about 19 percent.

Where to get antioxidants

A variety of foods can provide you with the antioxidants you need for good eye health.

Vitamin E. Good sources of vitamin E include vegetable oils and products made from them. Wheat germ, nuts and avocados also contain relatively high amounts.

Vitamin C. Good sources of vitamin C include green and red peppers, collard greens, broccoli, spinach, tomatoes, potatoes, strawberries and other berries, oranges, grapefruits and other citrus fruits.

Carotenoids. Good sources of carotenoids include deep yellow, dark green and red vegetables and fruits, including carrots, winter squash, sweet potatoes, broccoli, bell peppers, tomatoes, papayas, cantaloupe, mangoes, apricots and watermelon. Beta carotene is the best-known carotenoid but not the only one. Lutein and zeaxanthin are found in dark green leafy vegetables, including spinach, kale, collard greens, mustard greens, Swiss chard, watercress and parsley. Red peppers and romaine lettuce contain smaller amounts of these two carotenoids.

Some key points: Only participants in the intermediate and advanced stages of macular degeneration benefited from the supplements. Participants with no AMD or in the early stages of the disease did not. The supplements had no effect on preventing cataracts, as had been hoped.

The antioxidant combination also raised several concerns during the course of the study. For example, smokers or recent nonsmokers began experiencing side effects from the large doses of beta carotene.

The formulation used in the study is marketed as Ocuvite PreserVision and can be purchased at local pharmacies. Other manufactured products claim to be similar to the AREDS formulation, but make sure to check the dosage. If you take high doses of the ingredients in the formulation separately, don't omit some while including others. You should also see your eye doctor regularly during the course of treatment.

High-dose combinations of antioxidants should only be used for what clinical trials such as AREDS have shown them to be effective for — preventing intermediate or advanced macular degeneration from progressing to a more advanced stage. At this point, there's little evidence that the AREDS formulation can prevent macular degeneration, even among those with a family history of the disease.

The AREDS formulation

The daily supplements used in the Age-Related Eye Disease Study contained a combination of the following vitamins and minerals:

Vitamin C . . . . 500 milligrams (mg)
Vitamin E . . . . 400 international units (IU)
Beta carotene . . . . 15 mg (often as vitamin A — up to 25,000 IU)
Zinc . . . . 80 mg (as zinc oxide)
Copper . . . . 2 mg (as cupric oxide)

Lutein and zeaxanthin. In addition to the nutrients used in AREDS, scientists are interested in the roles that lutein and zeaxanthin may play in the prevention of macular degeneration. One of the primary functions of these two carotenoids, which are highly concentrated in the macula, is believed to be filtering out damaging radiation from sunlight. Both substances also have strong antioxidant qualities. Dietary sources of lutein and zeaxanthin include dark green leafy vegetables.

A randomized trial called AREDS 2 has been set up to study the effects of a high-dose combination of lutein, zeaxanthin and omega-3 fatty acids on the development of macular degeneration and cataracts. If study results turn out positive, scientists may consider eliminating beta carotene and zinc from the original AREDS formulation, both of which caused certain negative effects.

Other antioxidants. It will likely take many more years of careful research to determine the benefits of other antioxidants to your eye health. And don't take everything you hear at face value. For example, anthocyanin, an antioxidant found in blueberries and bilberries, has long been promoted for a variety of eye disorders, ranging from nearsightedness and poor night vision to cataracts, glaucoma and macular degeneration. Although preclinical trials have shown promise, there's still insufficient evidence from well-designed studies and, in fact, certain findings have contradicted the claims.

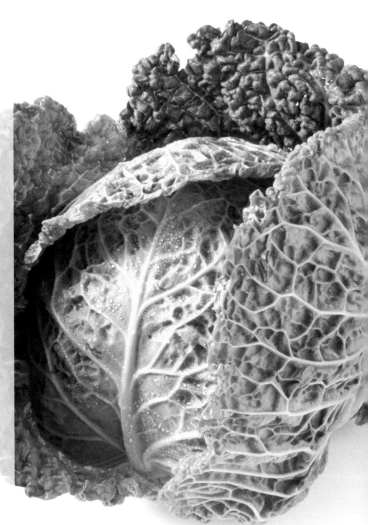

Multivitamins

Observational studies indicate that multivitamins may lower the risk of cataracts, but these findings haven't been confirmed with randomized controlled clinical trials. It's entirely possible that the lower risk could be due to another factor of healthy living practiced by the people taking the vitamins. And although multivitamins may help ensure an adequate amount of nutrients to the retina, there's no evidence that they slow the progression of macular degeneration. Keep in mind that megadoses of vitamins can have dangerous side effects so, unless advised by your doctor, stick to the recommended daily requirement listed on the bottle.

Zinc

Zinc is one of the most common trace minerals in your body and highly concentrated in the retina. Although it's not known exactly what role zinc plays in eye function, some scientists speculate that lack of zinc may contribute to macular degeneration. Others believe that zinc may offer some protection against inflammation and age-related damage to the retina. A diet with plenty of fruits and veg-etables usually provides you with an adequate amount of zinc, but there remains some interest in studying the long-term effect of zinc supplements. There are dangers with high doses of this mineral, as demonstrated with the AREDS formulation, because zinc may reduce copper or iron absorption into the bloodstream. In addition, excess zinc in your system isn't as easy to flush out of the body as are water-soluble vitamins.

Red wine

Many people who enjoy an occasional glass of wine have been heartened in recent years by studies proclaiming the health benefits of such practice. Results from studies such as the Reykjavik Eye Study indicate that, while nondrinkers and heavy drinkers of any type of alcohol have an increased risk of cataracts, moderate drinkers of red wine may have about half the risk. Moderate drinking is loosely defined as being anywhere from two to three glasses a day to around two glasses a month. Moderate drinking of beer and hard liquor doesn't appear to have the same positive effects. While continuing to analyze the data, scientists wish to avoid generalizing about cataracts too much, as cortical cataracts and nuclear cataracts often can develop in response to very different factors.

Sticking with the basics

The most eye-friendly diet is a healthy, balanced diet that you regularly eat. With a well-balanced diet, your eyes should get all of the nutrients they need. It's fine to take a daily vitamin and mineral supplement, but remember that supplements aren't a substitute for eating a variety of healthy foods.

To date, study results show that certain combinations of vitamins and minerals may potentially help slow or stop the progress of an eye disorder, but none appears to have a significant effect on people with no existing vision problems.

Keep in mind that the supplements used in these studies have been extremely high doses, beyond what you can get in your regular diet. If you're taking one of these supplements, be alert for negative side effects, especially if you're taking other prescription or over-the-counter medications.

Reducing your risk of eye disease through diet doesn't happen overnight. It likely involves years of good nutrition. Does that mean it may be too late for you to benefit from increasing the amount of antioxidants in your diet? Absolutely not. Eating more vegetables and fruits certainly won't hurt you. And on the chance that they might protect your eyesight, enjoy spinach, tomatoes and other fresh produce each day.

At a glance

Common eye conditions

Many common eye conditions are bothersome, but they don't cause serious or permanent damage to your sight. Your eyes may become red, itchy, irritated, and teary or dry — no fun, to be sure. However, with proper care, you should be able to ease the symptoms and maintain clear, comfortable vision. Though these conditions may involve a doctor visit, for the most part, they require active steps at home to treat the problem and prevent a recurrence. Some of the most common eye problems are described in this section, along with guidelines for treatment.

Painful, itchy or irritated eyes

Conjunctivitis

Persistent redness in an eye, especially if it's accompanied by irritation or pain, may signal an inflammation known as conjunctivitis (kun-junk-tih-VI-tis), commonly called pink eye.

A virus, bacterium or allergic reaction may cause conjunctivitis. Viral and bacterial conjunctivitis are extremely infectious and often associated with a cold or sore throat. Conjunctivitis caused by an allergic reaction stems from exposure to an allergen, a substance that irritates the eye.

All forms of conjunctivitis share common symptoms. Most noticeably, inflammation enlarges the small blood vessels of the conjunctiva, giving it a reddish or pinkish coloration (hyperemia) — hence the name "pink eye." Your eye may become itchy and teary. You may feel a scratchy sensation when you blink, as if fine grains of sand were lodged under the eyelids. You may wake up in the morning with your eyelids encrusted with discharge. You may experience blurred vision and be oversensitive to light.

Applying a compress may soothe discomfort in the affected eye. A warm compress works best for viral and bacterial conjunctivitis, but a cold compress helps relieve the itching of allergic conjunctivitis. Soak a clean cloth in water, squeeze it dry and lay it over your closed eyelids for 10 minutes.

Viral conjunctivitis

Viral conjunctivitis typically spreads through contact with contaminated tears or nasal fluids. Symptoms usually appear seven to 10 days after you've been infected. It produces a watery or mucous discharge. Often infection in one eye leads to that in the other. Unfortunately, you must wait for viral conjunctivitis to run its course and go away on its own — which may take up to two or three weeks.

Bacterial conjunctivitis

Bacterial conjunctivitis produces a sticky, yellow-green discharge that's thicker than the discharge from viral conjunctivitis. When you wake up in the morning, your eyes may be matted shut by crusty discharge. The infection often starts in one eye and spreads to the other.

The bacteria that cause conjunctivitis can be contracted from many sources, including another bacterial infection. Germs are passed from person to person through infected body fluids or by hand-to-eye contact. Treatment with antibiotics should clear the infection within seven days.

Stopping the spread

Good hygiene is essential for controlling the spread of conjunctivitis.
- Keep your hands away from your eyes.
- Wash your hands frequently.
- Dispose of tissues after use.
- Don't share towels, washcloths, pillowcases, handkerchiefs, contact lenses, lens cleaning solution or eyedrops with another person.
- If you have conjunctivitis, stay home from work, school or activities until you have no discharge from your eyes.
- Dispose of mascara and purchase new when the infection is gone.

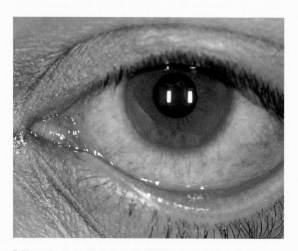

Viral conjunctivitis
Viral infection of the conjunctiva engorges blood vessels of the eye, giving it a swollen, red and teary appearance.

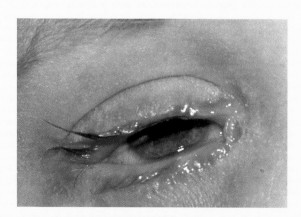

Bacterial conjunctivitis
Bacterial conjunctivitis not only causes redness and swelling but also often produces a thicker mucous discharge than does viral conjunctivitis.

Painful, itchy or irritated eyes

Allergic conjunctivitis

Allergic conjunctivitis is not an infection. Rather it's a response to an allergen — a substance that irritates your body. What may be an allergen for you may have little or no effect on another person. Common allergens include pollen, dust, mold, animal dander and skin, chemicals in common household products, spray perfumes and certain medications. Your body reacts to the allergen by releasing chemicals, such as histamine, that cause allergy symptoms.

Allergic conjunctivitis, like the viral and bacterial forms, can make your eyes red and itchy. A ropy discharge may form, particularly after rubbing your eyes. Other symptoms may include intense tearing, a runny nose and sneezing. The condition often affects both eyes at once.

Depending on the allergic trigger, treatment may clear up the inflammation quickly or it may only ease the discomfort. For example, conjunctivitis caused by hay fever can last a whole season and return every year.

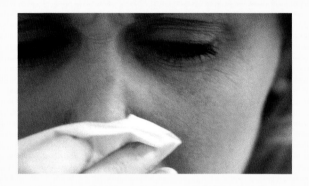

Eyedrops and oral medications that may help relieve allergy symptoms include:

- **Decongestants** that contain chemicals to reduce eye redness, along with relieving congestion. Most are available over-the-counter, and some are combined with an antihistamine. Prolonged use may have a "rebound effect," causing increased swelling and redness. Don't use decongestant eyedrops if you have glaucoma.
- **Antihistamines** block the action of histamine, the chemical released by your immune system that's responsible for many allergy symptoms. Antihistamine medications may be prescription or over-the-counter.
- **Nonsteroidal anti-inflammatory drugs (NSAIDs)**, such as aspirin and ibuprofen (Advil, Motrin, others)

may help relieve inflammation and swelling.

- **Mast cell stabilizers** affect certain cells in the eye (mast cells) that release histamine and other chemicals that cause allergy symptoms. They function best when used before exposure to the allergen. Some drops combine antihistamine and mast cell stabilizers.
- **Corticosteroid eyedrops** may be prescribed if antihistamine and decongestant medications fail to relieve allergy symptoms. These potent medications should only be used as prescribed by your doctor because prolonged use can increase your risk of glaucoma, cataracts and eye infection.

One of the best ways to deal with allergic conjunctivitis is to avoid those allergens that trigger your symptoms — although sometimes that's difficult to do. If you're allergic to pollen, for example, and pollen counts are high, try to stay indoors, keep your doors and windows closed, and use an air conditioner. If you're allergic to animal dander, you may need to avoid pets that shed hair. If a chemical in your contact lens solution causes an allergic reaction, try switching brands or wearing glasses.

Other allergic reactions

Some allergic reactions can be a source of discomfort without necessarily reddening the eye. This type of reaction is sometimes due to substances that are not true allergens, such as cigarette smoke, perfume and exhaust fumes. Your eyes may become irritated, itchy and watery. The eyelids may become puffy, and dark circles may appear under your eyes. Scaly, red skin may appear around the eye. You might be tempted to rub your eyes, but doing so just causes more irritation.

Treatment for this type of reaction is the same as that for allergic conjunctivitis. For many people, an antihistamine provides sufficient relief. Applying a cold compress several times a day may decrease swelling around the eye. In severe cases, your doctor may prescribe medication, such as a steroid cream or ointment. Applying a steroid near the eye involves risk and should be used exactly as prescribed.

Scleritis and episcleritis

The sclera is the layer of tissue that forms the wall of the eyeball — the white of the eye. Sandwiched between the sclera and the outer membrane (conjunctiva) is a transparent tissue called the episclera. Occasionally, the sclera or episclera becomes inflamed. Both conditions are characterized by patchy redness and swelling in the eye. Scleritis may be accompanied by dull pain and blurred vision.

Episcleritis is a mild inflammation that generally disappears on its own after a week or two. Scleritis is a less common but more serious disorder, often associated with inflammatory bowel disease or rheumatoid arthritis. It commonly affects people between the ages of 30 and 60. Steroids in drop or ointment form may help reduce the inflammation. Oral anti-inflammatory drugs, such as ibuprofen, or oral steroids also may be used.

Uveitis

The uvea is a layer of tissue between the retina and sclera, which includes the choroid, iris and ciliary body. Inflammation of the uvea is called uveitis (u-vee-I-tis). When the inflammation affects primarily the iris, the condition is called iritis (i-RI-tis). Signs and symptoms may appear suddenly and include eye pain and redness, blurred vision, floaters and sensitivity to light.

The condition is associated with disorders such as rheumatoid arthritis or inflammatory bowel disease, infections such as syphilis or tuberculosis, eye injury and certain cancers. Left untreated, uveitis can cause permanent eye damage. Besides vision loss, complications may include glaucoma, cataract, and retinal and optic nerve damage.

Your doctor may treat uveitis with anti-inflammatory drugs, often in the form of eyedrops. Oral steroids may be prescribed for more severe cases. A dilating drug also may be prescribed that "freezes" the iris and prevents it from moving, lessening the chance of scarring. If the condition is caused by an infection, antibiotics or other medications may be prescribed. If the uveitis is caused by an underlying condition, treatment will focus on that condition.

Corneal abrasion or injury

As the most exposed part of the eye, the cornea is susceptible to injuries and infections. The most common corneal injury is an abrasion caused by scratching or rubbing. This can happen when a speck of sand scratches the surface or if you wear your contact lenses for too long. Without proper eye protection, your cornea can also be burned by ultraviolet radiation from the sun, a sunlamp or a welding arc.

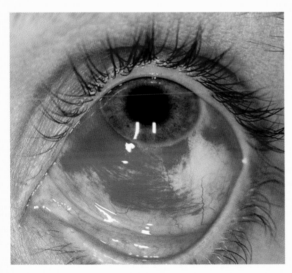

Subconjunctival hemorrhage
The condition occurs when a small blood vessel in the eye breaks. It may look scary, but the condition is harmless and usually disappears in a few days.

Following a corneal injury, the tissue around your eye may swell and the eye itself may redden and hurt intensely. You may blink more than usual. Some people don't feel symptoms for several hours after the injury, and then find themselves in extreme discomfort.

Simple corneal abrasions are treated by removing any foreign material, then allowing the eye to heal itself — often within a day or two. Your doctor may apply an antibiotic ointment or drops to prevent infection and prescribe a pain reliever. More serious injury to the cornea may require surgical treatment.

Subconjunctival bleeding

A bright red patch on the white of your eye can be alarming. This spot is usually a subconjunctival hemorrhage. It happens when a blood vessel in the conjunctiva breaks after you cough, sneeze or vomit forcefully — but often there's no identifiable reason at all. Eye trauma also can cause a hemorrhage. If you have pain with a broken blood vessel or if you get them recurrently, contact your doctor. Otherwise, the condition should improve on its own.

Sty

A sty is a red lump on the edge of your eyelid that may resemble a boil or pimple. It stems from a bacterial infection around the root of an eyelash. A sty, which develops gradually over several days, is usually harmless to the eye but fills with pus and becomes painful to touch. You may get more than one sty at a time because the bacteria that infect one hair follicle can spread and infect other follicles.

About one week after a sty appears it usually ruptures, which relieves the

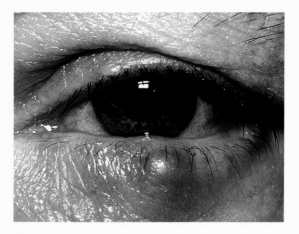

Sty

A sty is a painful reddish swelling caused by a bacterial infection along the edge of your eyelid.

pain. The swelling goes down in another week or so. Begin using a warm compress as soon as you feel a sty coming on. Apply the compress four times a day for 10 minutes until the sty opens. Don't squeeze the sty in an effort to remove the pus — let it burst on its own. Once the sty has opened, wash your eyelid thoroughly to prevent the bacteria from spreading.

Consult your doctor if the sty interferes with your vision or doesn't disappear on its own. A stubborn sty may need to be lanced and drained. If you're prone to recurring sties, your doctor may prescribe antibiotic treatment.

Chalazion

Another form of swelling on the eyelid is a chalazion (sha-LA-zee-on). Unlike a sty, it's relatively painless and develops away from the eyelid edge. A chalazion is not an infection. Rather, it's a swelling caused by blockage of a small oil gland in the eyelid. Bacteria may grow within the blocked gland.

A chalazion will often go away without treatment, although how long that takes may vary from one to two months. Applying a warm compress to the area four times a day for 10 minutes may help. You can also massage the area to try and break up the lump. If the chalazion gets big enough to affect your vision, your doctor may prescribe an antibiotic ointment. If this treatment is unsuccessful or if the swelling continues to enlarge, your doctor may need to drain the chalazion surgically.

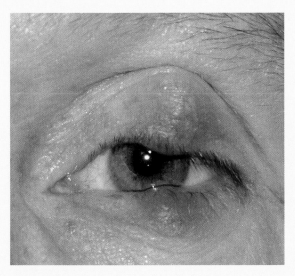

Chalazion

A chalazion (on the upper eyelid) is a relatively painless swelling caused by inflammation, usually located away from the edge of your eyelid. (A sty is located on the lower eyelid.)

Twitchy eyelids

From time to time your eyelid may take on a life of its own. This involuntary twitching usually lasts only a few seconds, but it can be recurrent and irritating and make you wonder if something's wrong with your eye.

A twitch is usually considered harmless. Eye twitches are similar to the occasional muscle twitch in a hand, forearm, leg or foot. No one knows exactly what causes these flutters, although they're often associated with fatigue or stress. Very rarely, a twitching eyelid is a symptom of a muscle or nerve disease, but this type of fluctuation tends to be distinct from the common eye twitch.

You may relieve the twitching by gently massaging the affected eyelid. To do this, move your index finger back and forth from the inner to the outer part of the lid for approximately one minute. Use the same amount of pressure that you put on a computer keyboard. Massage may be more effective if you use a warm compress on the eyelid for about 10 minutes beforehand.

Blepharitis

Blepharitis (blef-uh-RI-tis) is an inflammation of the eyelids along the lid margins where the eyelashes grow. Commonly, blepharitis occurs when tiny oil glands located at the base of the eyelashes malfunction. The oil excess encourages the growth of bacteria, which can make the eyelids irritated and itchy. Although it may feel uncomfortable and unattractive, blepharitis doesn't cause permanent damage to your eyesight.

Signs and symptoms of blepharitis also include watery or red eyes, a gritty sensation in the eyes, burning or swollen eyelids, sensitivity to light, frothy tears, and flaking skin around the eyes. The eyelids appear greasy and crusted with scales that cling to the lashes and cause the eyelids to stick together at night. Don't be too concerned if you have to pry your eyes open in the morning because of these sticky secretions. Sometimes, you may notice only the presence of dried tear secretions in the morning that feel like small grains of sand.

Blepharitis may be caused by a combination of factors other than malfunctioning oil glands in your eyelid. Conditions

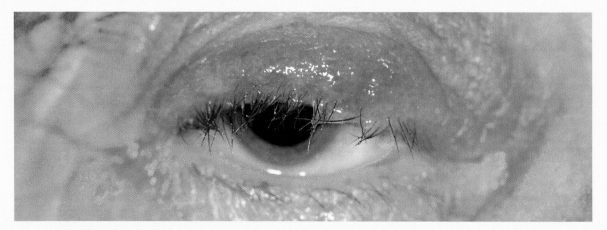

Blepharitis

An eyelid with blepharitis may appear red and swollen with scaly, greasy debris along the lid margin. Blepharitis is often associated with dandruff of the scalp and the eyebrows.

Eyelid-related problems

associated with blepharitis include seborrheic dermatitis (dandruff of the scalp and eyebrows) and rosacea (a skin condition characterized by facial redness). Possible complications of blepharitis include the loss of eyelashes, abnormal eyelash growth, a sty, chalazion, excess tearing or dry eyes, chronic pink eye, and injury to the cornea.

Blepharitis can be difficult to treat. The key is good hygiene, which may allow you to control the symptoms. Follow this remedy once or twice a day:

1. Apply a warm compress over your closed eyes for approximately 10 minutes.
2. Immediately afterward, use a washcloth moistened with warm water and a few drops of baby shampoo to wash away oily debris at the base of the eyelashes. To do this, gently pull the eyelid away from the eye to avoid accidental injury to the cornea from your washcloth.
3. Rinse the eyelids with warm water and gently pat them dry with a clean, dry towel. Ask your doctor about using a topical antibacterial solution after cleaning the eyelid in this manner.

Continue treatment until your symptoms disappear. Although you may be able to decrease the frequency of this cleaning, you should maintain an eyelid care routine to prevent a recurrence. If the condition doesn't improve with regular cleaning, contact your doctor. He or she may prescribe an antibiotic cream or ointment. In severe cases, eyedrops containing antibiotics and corticosteroids may be prescribed.

Itchy eyelids

Itchiness around the eyes often accompanies seasonal allergies, but it may also indicate contact dermatitis, an inflammation that results from your fingers coming in contact with an irritating substance and then touching your eyelids. Cosmetics also may cause allergic reactions to the sensitive skin around your eyes.

If your eyelids itch, don't rub or scratch them excessively. Rubbing ultimately can result in eczema, with persistent itching and scaling. If your eyelids are sensitive to certain cosmetics or other materials, avoid using them.

Entropion and ectropion

Sometimes, the eyelid — usually the lower lid — turns in toward the eye, allowing the eyelid and eyelashes to rub against the surface of the eye. Doctors refer to this condition as entropion. In addition to eye irritation, entropion causes excessive tearing, redness, discharge, crusting of the eyelid and a feeling that something is lodged in the eye. In severe cases, the turned-in lashes may scratch the cornea, resulting in infection.

Most often, entropion develops when the tissues of the eyelid weaken because of aging. An early sign of the condition is eye irritation in the morning, which usually clears during the day. The irritation usually becomes more frequent, even constant.

Ectropion — an inverse condition to entropion — describes the sagging and turning out of the lower eyelid. As a result, the eyelids can no longer close properly. Without adequate protection, the surface of the eye becomes dry and inflamed. Tears pool

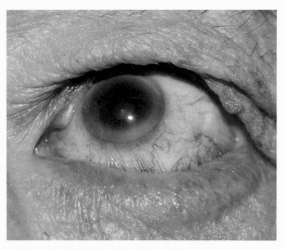 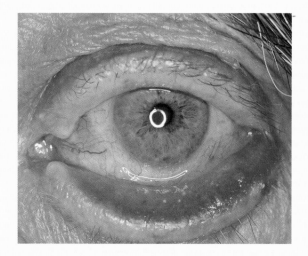

Entropion and ectropion
With entropion (left) the eyelid turns inward, allowing the lashes to rub against and irritate the eyeball. With ectropion (right) the eyelid sags away from the eyeball. Lacking protection and sufficient lubrication, the eye becomes red and irritated.

Eyelid-related problems

in the corners of the eyes and overflow onto your eyelids. Rubbing the eye leads to further irritation.

Like entropion, ectropion is most often due to age-related weakening of eyelid tissue. The condition may also stem from a facial nerve disorder, trauma, tumors or previous eyelid surgery. Sometimes, it may be associated with an underlying condition such as atopic dermatitis or lupus. Untreated ectropion may lead to eye infection and corneal damage.

Artificial tears or an ointment may offer temporary relief for either condition. Some people wear an eye shield at night to retain moisture. Others apply transparent adhesive tape to the skin of the eyelid near the lashes before sleep to help hold the lid in place.

The primary means of treating entropion and ectropion is surgery to reposition the eyelids. This simple procedure is performed on an outpatient basis using a local anesthetic. After surgery, you may wear an eye patch overnight and apply an antibiotic ointment for about a week.

Dermatochalasis

With age, your eyelid skin may begin to stretch and sag due to an accumulation of fat and to loss of muscle elasticity. This condition, called dermatochalasis (der-muh-toe-KAL-uh-sis), usually affects both eyes. Occasionally, the skin of your upper eyelids may sag over your eyelashes and interfere with your vision. The lower eyelids may form what are commonly referred to as bags under the eyes.

A surgical procedure called blepharoplasty (BLEF-uh-ro-plas-tee) may be performed to remove excess skin, muscle and fat from the eyelid. It's generally safe and can be done on an outpatient basis. Swelling or tenderness you may experience afterward should subside within two to four weeks. Mild cases are sometimes treated with laser surgery. In this procedure, the high-powered laser beam shrinks and tightens the tissue without removing it.

Whether your health insurer will pay for surgery depends on whether the condition impairs your vision.

Ptosis

Ptosis (TOE-sis) is a condition caused by a weakness of the eye muscle that raises the upper eyelid and keeps it in an open position. Whereas derma-tochalasis results in sagging eyelid skin, ptosis causes the entire eyelid to droop.

Ptosis often runs in families and can affect one or both eyes. Some children are born with the condition — usually in just one eye. In adults, ptosis may be a result of aging or injury, or a condition affecting nerve and muscle response, such as myasthenia gravis, diabetes or a brain tumor. A drooping eyelid that develops suddenly requires immediate attention because it may be the sign of a stroke or another acute problem.

If the drooping eyelid doesn't affect your vision and you're not bothered by its appearance, your doctor may not treat the condition. If the drooping eyelid has reduced your vision, a thorough eye examination may be necessary to determine the cause. If the droop is due to a nerve or muscle condition, treating the underlying cause may improve ptosis. If the drooping is a result of aging or injury, your doctor may recommend surgery to strengthen the muscle and lift the lid. This is a complicated operation that should be performed by a specialist.

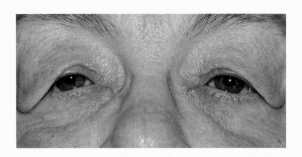

Dermatochalasis
A relaxation of the skin of the upper eyelid may cause it to droop over the eyelashes and interfere with your vision.

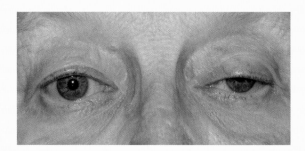

Ptosis
A weakened muscle that raises the upper eyelid can cause the entire lid to droop over the eye (in this case, the left eye).

Tear-related problems

Healthy eyes are covered by a thin tear film — a layer that keeps the surface of the eyes moist without any fluid overflowing the eyelids. The tear glands, also called the lacrimal glands, are located underneath the skin of the upper eyelids. Glands along the edges of the eyelids also produce some tear components. Tears get to the eye through openings in the upper eyelids. When you blink, your eyelids spread the fluid across the surface of your eyes and sweep excess tears into tear ducts (lacrimal ducts) that drain to your nose — that's why your nose often runs when you cry. Basic tearing occurs at a steady rate to prevent dry eyes and to maintain clear vision.

Reflex tearing produces a large quantity of fluid in response to sudden eye irritation or to strong emotions, often causing tears to overflow. For example, when your eyes are affected by dust or smoke, extra tears form to wash away the foreign material. A sad movie or a joyous wedding also can make tears stream down your cheeks. There are other causes of teary eyes, including allergic reaction, sinus infection, eye infection and nasal problems.

Occasionally, tear duct problems result in continuously watering eyes.

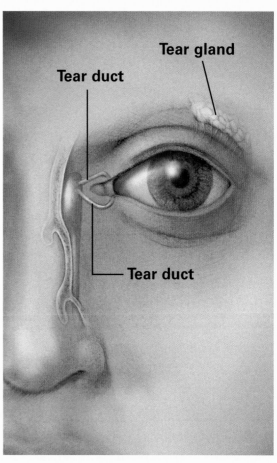

The tear system
The tear gland, located in the upper eyelid, continuously supplies fluid that's spread across the surface of your eye by the blinking action of your eyelids. Excess fluid is swept to the tear ducts and drains into your nose.

Dry eyes

Tear production tends to decrease as you get older, and decreased production can destabilize the tear film and create dry spots on the cornea that cause irritation and reduce vision. Some people produce a normal amount of tears, but the composition of the tears is of poor quality. The tears lack essential components for eye lubrication. Problems with the eyelids can also cause dryness.

Tear quality

Tears are more than just water. They're a complex mixture that also includes fatty oils, proteins, electrolytes and bacteria-fighting substances. This mixture helps make the eye surface smooth and clear. The tear film has three basic layers:

- **Mucus.** The inner layer, which consists of mucus, allows tears to spread evenly over the surface of the eye.
- **Water.** The middle layer is mostly water with a little bit of salt. It cleanses the eye and washes away foreign irritants.
- **Oil.** The outer layer, produced by glands on the edge of the eyelid, contains fatty oils. The oil smooths the tear surface and slows the evaporation of the watery layer.

Sometimes, this mix of ingredients is off-balance, which causes the tears to evaporate too fast. Certain diseases also can change the oil and mucus layers of your tears. Some skin disorders can disrupt production of the oil layer.

The medical term for dry eyes is keratoconjunctivitis sicca (ker-uh-to-kun-junk-ti-VIE-tis SIK-uh). Signs and symptoms include a stinging, burning, or scratchy sensation, swelling and redness, and stringy mucus in or around the eyes. Eye fatigue and sensitivity to light are increased. The condition usually affects both eyes. It's most common among women following menopause, perhaps due to hormonal changes. Dry eyes are also associated with certain medical conditions such as rheumatoid arthritis and Sjogren's syndrome.

Although dry eyes don't usually cause vision damage, the condition often prompts people to seek treatment.

Tear-related problems

If my eyes are dry, why are they watering?

It may sound like a contradiction, but it's possible to have dry eyes and still have tears streaming down your cheeks. When your eyes become irritated from dryness, the tear glands respond by flooding the eyes with reflex tears. Because reflex tears contain more water and less oil than basic tears do, they evaporate faster and don't help the dryness. However, the excess fluid often overwhelms the tear ducts and overflows your eyelids.

If your eyes feel dry and irritated, your eye doctor can test both the quantity and quality of your tears. He or she may measure your tear production using the Schirmer tear test. In this test, blotting strips of paper are placed under the lower eyelids. After five minutes your doctor measures the amount of strip soaked by your tears. Other tests use special dyes in eyedrops to determine the surface condition of your eye. The doctor looks for staining patterns on the cornea and measures the amount of time it takes before your tears evaporate.

The goal of treatment is to restore a more normal tear film and minimize the consequences of dryness:

- **Adding tears.** A mild case of dry eyes usually can be treated with artificial tears — use the lubricating drops as often as needed to provide relief. Preservative-free eyedrops may be the best choice.

- **Conserving tears.** Steps can be taken to retain tears by partially or completely closing your tear ducts with tiny silicone plugs, which can be removed at any time. In a more permanent option, a doctor numbs the area with an anesthetic and then applies a hot wire that shrinks the tissue, causing scarring that closes the tear duct.

- **Medications.** The only medication approved for chronic dry eyes is cyclosporine (Restasis). It decreases inflammation and helps increase the production of tears. Some people experience a burning sensation in their eyes when using the drug.

Common eye conditions
Tear-related problems

Like any liquid, tears evaporate when exposed to air. Here are some simple steps to help slow the evaporation:

- Avoid air blowing in your eyes from hair dryers, air conditioners or fans.
- Wear glasses on windy days and goggles while swimming.
- Keep your home humidity between 30 percent and 50 percent.
- Avoid rubbing your eyes, which may cause further irritation.
- Remember to blink. Blinking helps spread your tears more evenly.

Overflowing tears

Overflowing tears occur mostly among older adults and are associated with aging or injury to the nose. Too much tearing can result from excessive tear production due to an eye abrasion, infection of the eyelid, inward-growing eyelashes, allergies or nasal problems. When this happens, fluid backs up and spills over the eyelid, causing tears to run down your cheeks. Excessive tearing can also result from inadequate drainage through the tear ducts. A tear duct can become blocked by infection or by small particles of dirt or loose skin cells lodged in the duct.

See your doctor if your eye tears constantly over a period of several days. If the problem is a blocked duct, he or she may flush (irrigate) the tear duct in a simple outpatient procedure.

Infected tear duct

Occasionally, a tear duct can become infected from bacteria in stagnant tears. This is called dacryocystitis (dak-ree-o-sis-TI-tis). When it happens, the tissue between the eye and the bridge of the nose becomes swollen, red and tender. Tears can no longer make their way into the nose, causing an excessive amount of tearing.

Your doctor may prescribe an antibiotic for the infection. Applying a warm compress to the eye several times a day may help relieve discomfort.

If the symptoms are severe and don't improve, your doctor may recommend surgery to create a new tear duct. Thin silicone tubing is used to keep the new duct open while healing occurs. In rare cases, it's necessary to surgically implant an artificial tear duct. The artificial duct is made of unbreakable glass.

Chapter 8

Correcting vision

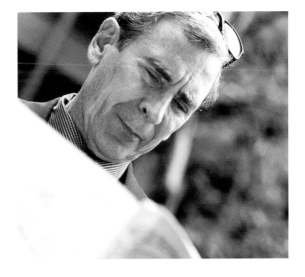

If you need sharper vision, eyeglasses and contact lenses provide many options for correcting common problems such as nearsightedness, farsightedness and astigmatism. A wide variety of styles and treatments are available to suit your lifestyle and fashion sense. If you prefer not having to deal with glasses or contact lenses, you may choose to have your vision corrected with an increasingly popular option — refractive surgery.

In deciding the best option for you, you and your eye doctor will consider your individual needs and preferences. The choice may narrow once you better understand the key differences among the various options.

Common vision problems

The intricate process of seeing, with so many complex interactions, can sometimes go wrong. The most common vision impairments are usually caused by a focusing problem of the cornea or lens or by an abnormal shape of the eye. These problems usually can be corrected with eyeglasses, contact lenses or surgery that adjusts the curvature of your cornea.

You see an object clearly when your cornea and lens have adjusted the point of focus so that a sharply defined image falls directly on your retina. If the focusing powers of your cornea and lens aren't coordinated with the length or the shape of your eye, however, the point of sharpest focus doesn't fall on the retina and the image you see is blurred.

Nearsightedness

If you're nearsighted — a condition called myopia (mi-O-pee-uh) — you can clearly see objects that are close to you, but objects farther away are blurry. Nearsightedness commonly occurs when your eye is slightly more elongated than normal. This causes light rays to be sharply focused in front of the retina instead of on the

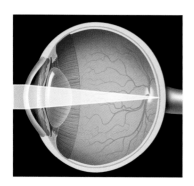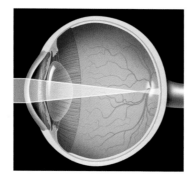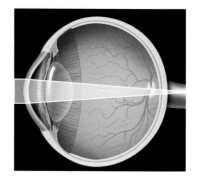

Common vision problems

With normal vision (left) the image is sharply focused on your retina. With nearsightedness (center) the point of sharpest focus lies in front of your retina, making distant objects appear blurry. With farsightedness (right) the point of sharpest focus falls behind your retina, making close-up objects appear blurry.

retina. Even with a normally shaped eye, you can be nearsighted if your cornea or lens is too steeply curved, bending light rays into focus before they reach the retina.

Many people first notice nearsightedness during childhood. Signs and symptoms include:

- Persistent squinting
- Sitting very close to a television or movie screen
- Holding books very close while reading
- Seeming to be unaware of distant objects

The condition affects boys and girls equally and tends to be hereditary. Vision problems may require new corrective lenses more than once a year, but then tend to stabilize during the young adult years.

Farsightedness

When you're farsighted — a condition called hyperopia (hi-pur-O-pee-uh) — you may see objects in the distance clearly but objects close to you are blurry. Very often, people are farsighted because their eye is shorter than normal, so the sharpest point of focus falls behind the retina. Far-

sightedness can also be caused by either a cornea or lens that's flattened, making refractive power weak.

Farsightedness is usually present at birth and tends to be hereditary. Most young people don't know they have the condition because the lenses of their eyes are very flexible and able to compensate for the condition. But as they grow older, the lenses become less elastic and unable to make the necessary adjustments. By middle age, most farsighted people need corrective lenses to improve near vision.

Signs and symptoms of farsightedness include:

- Nearby objects appearing blurry
- Needing to squint to see clearly
- Eyestrain, including burning eyes, aching in and around the eyes, and, rarely, a headache
- General eye and brow discomfort after prolonged reading

Astigmatism

Astigmatism (uh-STIG-muh-tiz-um) is a mild imperfection in the curvature of your eye that can blur vision. In a normal eye, the surface of the cornea or lens is curved evenly and smoothly in all directions. This allows

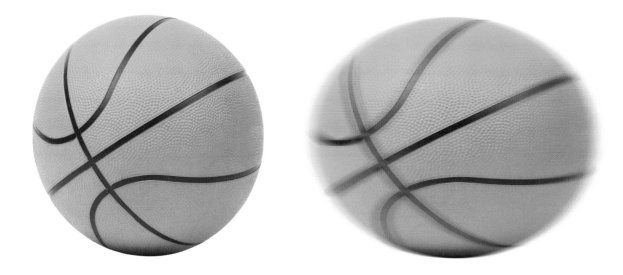

How astigmatism affects vision

Astigmatism is caused by the uneven curvature of your cornea or lens, which is unable to focus the light entering your eye, creating distorted, blurry vision. In this example, a round basketball (left) appears oblong (right) because the cornea is curved more sharply up and down than side to side.

for the ball that you're looking at, for example, to be perceived as round in shape.

Some people, however, have corneas and lenses, that have a slightly different surface curvature in one direction than in others — some areas are flatter or steeper than other areas. A round ball viewed through such a cornea or lens may be perceived as oblong, either horizontally, vertically or diagonally. This distortion of the image is astigmatism.

In most instances, astigmatism is inherited and usually established in early childhood, but sometimes it may develop after an injury or disease. It may occur in combination with nearsightedness or farsightedness. The condition generally remains constant and doesn't change throughout your life.

Astigmatism is common and often not pronounced enough to require corrective action. More serious astigmatism can be corrected with an eyeglass lens that counteracts the problem. This lens can be crafted to correct near-sightedness or farsightedness as well. Another option is refractive surgery.

Presbyopia

Although the term *presbyopia* (pres-be-O-pe-uh) may sound unfamiliar to many people, having the condition probably isn't unfamiliar for older adults. It refers to the gradual loss of the eye's ability to focus on nearby objects and is a natural part of aging. About the time you're 40 or older, you may notice that it's harder to read at the distance you're accustomed to. You're forced to hold the page farther away, sometimes at arm's length, to get the print in focus.

When you're young the lens in your eye is very elastic, giving you a wide range of focus. The lens naturally becomes thicker when you're doing close-up work so that the point of focus falls directly on your retina. As you get older, your lens hardens and gradually loses some of its elasticity, making it more difficult to focus on objects close to you. You may experience eyestrain and headaches from prolonged periods of reading, writing or sewing.

You can correct presbyopia with non-prescription or prescription reading glasses or contact lenses. The condition usually worsens with age, but by the time you are about age 65, the lenses in your eyes have lost most of their elasticity and don't change shape anymore. From this point on you're less likely to need changes in your prescription.

Poor color vision

People who have what's commonly known as colorblindness aren't really colorblind. That would mean they see only black and white. Actually, their problem is distinguishing between certain shades of color. Most people with poor color vision can't tell the difference between shades of red and green.

Poor color vision is usually inherited although eye diseases and certain medications also may cause it. The problem arises from chemical deficiencies in the cone cells. Defects can be mild, moderate or severe.

How corrective lenses work

Corrective lenses are custom-built lenses worn on or in front of your eyes that compensate for any problems with the shape of your eye or in the curvature of your cornea or lens. You may be more familiar with corrective lenses in the forms of eyeglasses, contact lenses and intraocular lenses. Using one of these resources helps resolve the refractive errors caused by nearsightedness, farsightedness, astigmatism and presbyopia.

The easiest way to explain a corrective lens is to think of it as a clear prism. Light passing through this prism will always bend (refract) toward the thickest part.

A concave (or minus) lens will be thickest at the edges, bending light outward. This kind of lens is used to correct nearsightedness by extending the point of focus inside the eye. A convex (or plus) lens is thickest in the middle, bending light inward. This lens is used to correct farsightedness.

The prescription you get from a routine eye exam includes the refractive

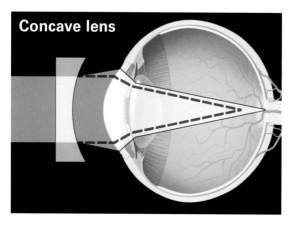
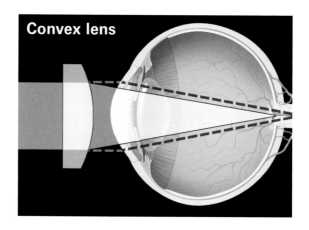

Basic lens shapes

A concave lens (left) corrects for nearsightedness. The dashed lines indicate where the point of focus would be without a corrective lens. A convex lens (right) corrects for farsightedness and is commonly used in reading glasses. The dashed lines indicate where the point of focus would be without a corrective lens.

Your eyeglasses prescription

Certain conventions and terminology are always used in a typical prescription for corrective lenses. The following example may help you understand your prescription:

	Sphere	Cylinder	Axis
OD	-2.75	2.25	90
OS	-1.75	2.00	90
		+1.50 add	

- **OD** (*oculus dexter*) is your right eye, identified on some prescriptions as RE.
- **OS** (*oculus sinister*) is your left eye, sometimes listed as LE.
- **Sphere** is the correction measurement for your nearsightedness or farsightedness.
- **Cylinder** is the correction measurement for astigmatism.
- **Axis** shows where the astigmatism correction should be on the lens — the position in degrees from horizontal. It can be anywhere from 1 to 180 degrees, with 90 degrees being a vertical (up-and-down) line.
- **+1.50 add** at the bottom of the chart indicates the need for an additional lens, in this case, bifocals for close-up work.

The numbers in the "Sphere" and "Cylinder" columns are units of lens power called diopters, which are based on how much bending (refraction) occurs when light passes through the lens. Diopters can increase or decrease in quarter (.25) increments. The higher the numbers in the prescription, the more refraction is necessary to correct your vision, and the thicker your lens.

The prescription in this example is for a person who is nearsighted with slight astigmatism. The diopters are preceded by a minus sign, meaning the lenses are concave. On a prescription to correct farsightedness, the numbers would be preceded by a plus sign, meaning the lenses are convex.

power needed to correct your vision problem. The higher the prescription numbers, the stronger the prescription. The prescription numbers identify the shape of the lens as convex, concave or — to correct astigmatism — cylindrical. The numbers also determine the thickness of the lens — the more light that must be refracted, the thicker the lens needs to be.

Eyeglasses

The variety of eyeglass styles and shapes can seem staggering. Thousands of frames and hundreds of lens designs are available. You can purchase eyeglasses from your eye doctor, small optical shop, department store, discount center, nationwide optical chain or on the Internet. When purchasing eyeglasses, there are a number of things you'll want to consider.

Lens materials

Eyeglass lenses are made of plastic or glass and, for the most part, either material can function as a suitable lens to correct your vision. The decision on which material to choose is

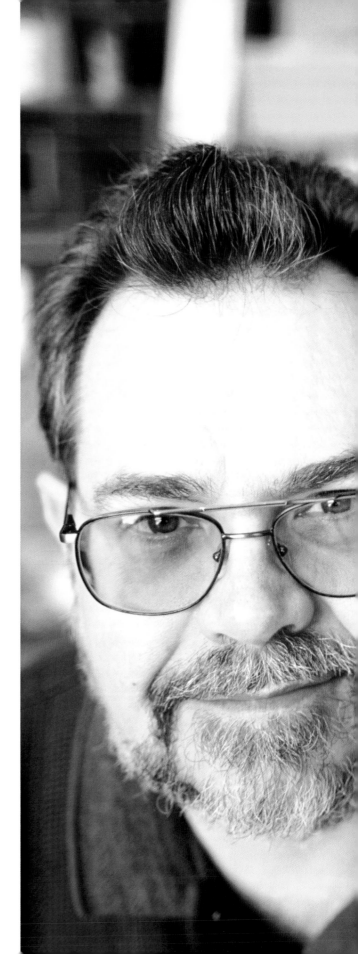

often based on factors of safety and lifestyle. A majority of eyeglass wearers choose plastic lenses, which tend to be lighter than glass lenses, but glass also has advantages.

Plastic. Lenses made with plastic are lightweight and more impact resistant than those made from glass. They're also easier to tint. Although they scratch more easily than do glass lenses, plastic lenses routinely come with a scratch-resistant coating. High-index plastic is a thin, lightweight option for moderate to strong prescriptions. Polycarbonate is the strongest plastic available and a preferred choice for active kids and for use in safety glasses. High-resin plastic will be a little thicker but considerably less expensive than high-index plastic.

Glass. Although glass lenses are more scratch resistant than are plastic lenses, they can be almost twice as heavy. For many people, the weight of glass lenses is a drawback — they're heavier than people are comfortable with. This is especially true for big frames. Another drawback to glass is that it can break or chip. However, glass may also provide the clearest possible vision.

Lens coatings

Scratch protection. A clear, hard coating is often applied to plastic lenses to make them more resistant to scratching. It's best that both sides of a lens are treated because you can easily scratch the inside surface while cleaning it. Scratch protection is often included in the cost but occasionally it's an additional charge.

Ultraviolet protection. Ultraviolet (UV) rays may contribute to age-related eye diseases such as cataracts and macular degeneration. High-index plastic and polycarbonate plastic lenses typically have UV protection included, so don't be talked into paying extra for UV protection that you may have already purchased.

Anti-reflection coating. Reflection and glare are bothersome, particularly if you have a stronger prescription, which increases glare. Anti-reflection (AR) coating helps block the light reflected off surfaces such as pavement, water, snow and glass. AR coating also reduces the light reflected off your lenses, making it useful if you're involved in public speaking or are often photographed.

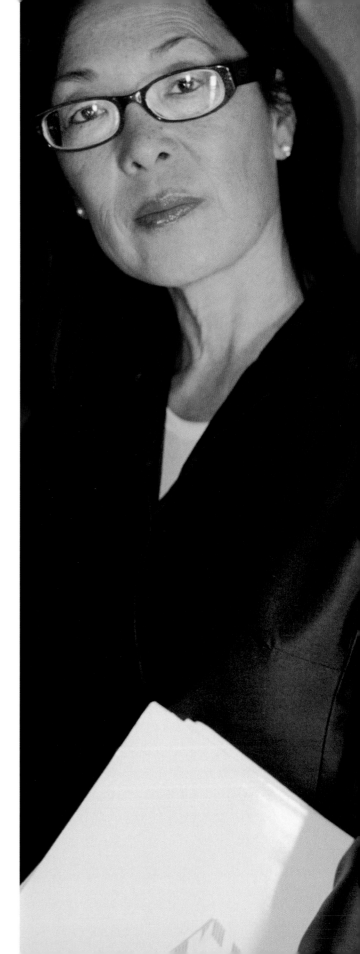

Lens treatments

Photochromatic. Photochromatic lenses are chemically treated to adjust to different levels of brightness. They get sunglass dark in direct sunlight and clear in a dimly lit room. Photochromatic lenses require UV light in order to change color, so they won't darken while you're driving because the windshield blocks these waves. You may need to keep a pair of sunglasses in the car.

Tint. Unlike photochromatic lenses, tinted lenses remain a constant shade in all levels of brightness. Adding color to your glasses can help if you're especially sensitive to light or simply want to make a fashion statement. Almost any color can be selected for a tint. Sunglasses are often gray or brown. A yellow tint can make objects appear sharper against a blue or green background.

Frames

When you're looking for new glasses, you may be tempted to start with the frames on a display rack. Save yourself time and guesswork by starting with your prescription. Some types of lenses work best with certain frames, and vice versa. For example, a prescription for astigmatism works well with small frames that have rounded edges — there's less distortion from having too much lens outside your line of vision. By reading your prescription, a skilled optician can help focus your search.

Size. The size of the frame can be important for your vision as well as your looks. Some eye doctors think the frame should cover 20 percent to 30 percent of your face, with the top of the frame following the line of your eyebrows. If your frame is too large, the lenses can pick up glare from overhead lights and distort your vision. If the frame is too small, your field of vision may be more limited than you'd like. If you need strong — and therefore thick — lenses, smaller frames can reduce the weight of your glasses.

Materials. Frames come in different grades of metal and plastic. Most often, you get what you pay for. If you buy the least expensive metal or plastic frame, you'll likely get a lower quality material — and depending on your needs and lifestyle, that may be just fine. Thin metal frames are often the lightest

and most stylish, but plastic frames are usually more durable and better able to support thick lenses.

The cheapest metal frames are made from a mixture of metals including nickel. Some frames may corrode from contact with perspiration and body oils. The more expensive metal frames made of titanium and carbon graphite are especially durable. And Flexon, a titanium-based alloy, has "shape memory." You can bend and twist it, and it springs back into shape.

Plastic frames also vary in their level of quality. Propionate plastic is used in the cheaper frames, zyl plastic is more stylish and colorful but can become brittle, and Kevlar, the same strong fiber used for military helmets, is very durable. Frames made of a resin called Optyl can be twisted around your finger and snap back into shape.

Fit. If your glasses fit correctly, they'll feel snug and secure, yet they won't rub behind your ears or irritate the bridge of your nose. If the frames bother you, they can be adjusted at the hinges, bridge or temples — the side arms of the frame that rest on your ears. You can also change the tilt of your glasses or adjust them closer to your face.

Your nose supports about 90 percent of the weight of your glasses. So the nose bridge is a major factor in how comfortable your glasses feel. The saddle bridge is a good choice for heavier glasses. It's a single piece of plastic molded to the frame that sits along the top and sides of your nose like a saddle, evenly spreading the weight of the lenses. The most common bridges are those with adjustable pads that sit on each side of your nose. They're flexible and easy to adjust, and the soft silicone material keeps the frames from sliding down your nose.

The temples should hook snugly around the ears and not be so thick that they block vision. Unlike standard hinges, which open to a set distance, flexible hinges can hold your glasses tightly to your head but allow the temples to be pulled wider so that the frames slip on or off easily.

It may take a period of a few days or even a week to get used to new glasses. During this time you may experience some eye ache, but it shouldn't be unbearable or persistent. If it's so painful that you can't wear the glasses, or if the pain lasts more than a week, check with the optician or your eye doctor. An adjustment to the frames may help. Also make sure that the prescription is correct. Regardless, it's a good idea to have the fit of your glasses checked every year or so. No matter how sturdy they are or how well you take care of them, glasses easily get out of alignment.

Bifocals, trifocals and progressive lenses

Many people have monofocal lenses. This means that their eyeglasses are equipped to correct just one form of vision deficiency: nearsightedness, farsightedness or astigmatism. Other people have multifocal lenses, which combine two or more focal powers in one lens. Chances are that by the time you enter your 40s, you may need to consider using one of these multifocal styles:

Bifocals. As the name implies, the bifocal style combines two focal powers in one lens. The top part of the lens provides your distance vision, while the lower part is equipped for your reading vision.

Trifocals. The trifocal lens adds a third power for an intermediate focus between your focus for distance and focus for reading. The added power helps you clearly see objects approximately two to four feet away, such as a computer monitor or items on a grocery store shelf.

Progressive. Unlike a trifocal lens, a progressive lens has no division lines separating the focal powers. Instead, the focal powers change smoothly as your eyes move from top to bottom. Some progressive lenses may distort vision along the bottom edge. However, newer lenses are being manufactured with less distortion.

It may take practice to adjust to multifocal lenses. The first step is to make sure the frames are properly adjusted to fit your head. Tilt your head up and down. Your line of vision should move smoothly from one focal power to the other in both eyes at precisely the same time.

Nonprescription reading glasses

As you enter your 40s, you may find that you need glasses for reading. Nonprescription reading glasses with

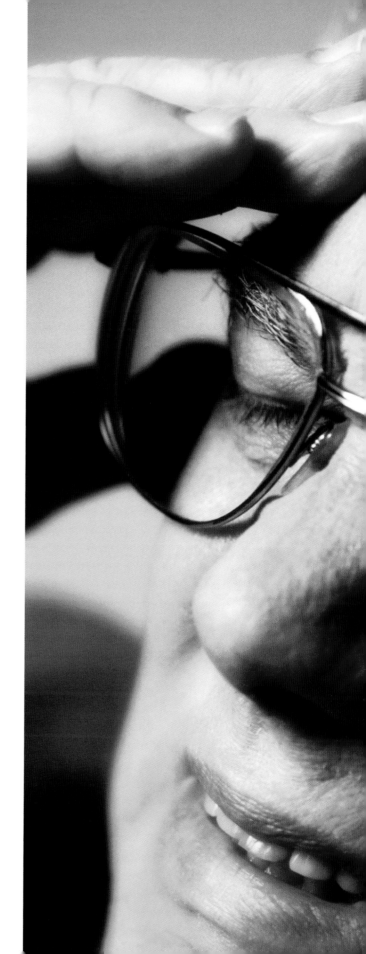

lenses of various strengths are commonly found in pharmacies and discount stores. Reading glasses may also function when worn over contact lenses that correct for distance vision.

If your eye doctor has told you the correction for your reading vision, look for lenses of that focal power. Otherwise, use trial and error by holding printed material about 14 to 16 inches from your eyes. When you find a pair of glasses that allows you to read comfortably, that's probably the power you need. This general guide shows which focal power is commonly associated with each of several age ranges:

Ages	Power
40 to 45	+1.25
46 to 50	+1.50
51 to 55	+1.75
56 to 60	+2.00
61 to 65	+2.25
Over 65	+2.50

Keep in mind that you'll need prescription reading glasses if each eye requires a different power. Whether you use prescription or nonprescription reading glasses, it's a good idea to see your eye doctor whenever you notice vision changes.

Contact lenses

For some people, glasses are a nuisance. They slide around on your nose. They attract dirt like a kid. They need windshield wipers when it rains. They fog up when you come in from the cold. And you're almost certain that someday a mishap is going to turn them into abstract artwork. Contact lenses are a nice alternative to glasses. Contacts are thin, clear disks of plastic that float on the tear film that coats your cornea. If you want to wear contacts, odds are you can. Most people interested in giving them a try are able to wear them.

Types of contact lenses

Contact lenses have come a long way since Leonardo da Vinci sketched a concept of them about 500 years ago, and since a German scientist in 1887 manufactured the first pair of contact lenses out of glass — which, by the way, the human eye couldn't tolerate. It wasn't until the coming of plastics in the 1940s that contacts became practical. Hard contacts developed at that time were well tolerated, and the type of plastic used in those lenses is still used today.

Hard lenses. Only a small percentage of contact wearers still use the original style of hard contacts. These lenses provide sharp vision, but they also block oxygen from passing through them to nourish your cornea. Hard lenses are also the most difficult contacts to get used to. Still, some people prefer hard lenses because they're durable. If you take good care of them, they can last a decade or more.

Rigid, gas permeable lenses. Unlike hard lenses, rigid, gas permeable lenses are slightly more flexible and more porous to oxygen. They're generally easier to adapt to and more comfortable than hard lenses. They may be a good choice for someone who, for example, has strong astigmatism. But "gas perms" have certain drawbacks, similar to hard lenses. You have to wear them regularly to get your eyes used to them. They can slip off the cornea and pop out of your eye. And it's easy for dust to get under them and irritate your eyes.

Soft contacts. Doctors sometimes call soft contacts "hydrogels" because these thin, flexible lenses hold water, which makes them soft and comfortable and allows them to conform to the shape of your eye. The water

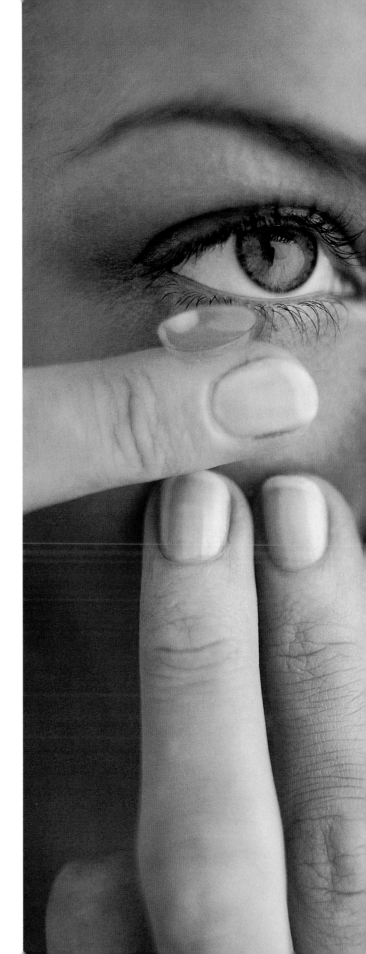

content varies from about one-third to three-fourths of the lens, depending on the material.

Unlike hard lenses, soft contacts allow oxygen to pass through the plastic and nourish your cornea. They also tend to stay in place on your eye, which makes them an excellent choice if you're active. But soft contacts aren't nearly as durable as hard contacts, and they can be torn if you handle them roughly. They also can't correct some common vision problems, such as a high degree of astigmatism. Several kinds of soft contacts are available:

Daily wear. As the name implies, daily wear, or conventional, contacts are designed to be worn when you're awake and to be removed before you go to sleep. They should not be kept in your eyes overnight. Due to microorganisms and surface buildup, you'll need to clean the lenses every day you wear them and replace them on a regular schedule.

Disposable wear. Disposable, or frequent-replacement, lenses are worn for a short time and then discarded. Some are replaced daily while others can be worn for a week or month before they're thrown away, depending on the design and material and how well you take care of them.

Disposable lenses are thinner and more porous to oxygen than daily wear lenses, making them even more comfortable. They may be a good choice if you have eye allergies.

Extended wear. Extended wear lenses are designed for up to seven days of wear without having to remove them. These lenses provide adequate oxygen to your cornea even while you're sleeping. Most eye doctors don't recommend extended wear lenses because, regardless of how well they're made, your eyes receive less oxygen when you wear contacts while sleeping. Furthermore, you're at greater risk of corneal infection because the buildup of bacteria on the lenses increases dramatically if you wear them overnight.

Lens options

To improve or fine-tune your vision, your eye doctor may recommend one of these contact lens options:

Bifocal. Bifocal contact lenses can have a reading and distance correction on each lens, like bifocal glasses. The reading section of each lens is weighted, so it stays at the bottom of your cornea and is available when you look down.

Monovision. With monovision contact lenses, the contact in one eye corrects for reading vision and the con-

tact in the other eye corrects for distance vision. Your brain typically adjusts to this unequal correction, but your vision may be a bit more blurry than normal.

Modified monovision. With this option, you wear a bifocal contact lens in your nondominant eye and a

Inside out?

Soft lenses sometimes turn inside out as you handle them. Putting them in your eye this way causes irritation and watering. In fact, if your eye hurts as soon as you insert a lens, it's very likely the contact is inside out.

There are two ways to check whether a contact is inside out before putting it in your eye. The first way is to hold the lens on the tip of your finger and look closely at the rim. If the rim is pointing straight up like the edge of a bowl, it's OK. If the edge is flared out, the lens is likely inside out.

A second way is to put the lens on a crease line in the palm of your hand and gently start to cup your hand. If the edges roll neatly toward each other, like they're forming a tiny taco shell, the lens is right side out. If they start to fold backward, away from the center, the lens is turned inside out.

contact lens for distance correction in your dominant eye. This allows you to use both eyes for distance, but only one for reading.

Proper lens care

Anytime you remove a contact lens from your eye, the lens should be cleaned before it's reinserted. Wearing a used lens that hasn't been cleaned greatly increases your risk of eye infection.

Most eye doctors will provide a starter cleaning kit with your new contact lenses. The kit usually contains instructions on how to proceed with the cleaning. These tips may also be helpful:

- Before handling the lenses, wash your hands with mild soap. Avoid creamy soaps, which leave a film on your hands that can transfer to the lenses. Rinse and dry your hands with a lint-free towel so that you don't get lint on the lens.
- Don't use water or saliva to clean your lenses. They contain microorganisms that can cause infection. (One particular organism, called acanthamoeba, can cause a sight-threatening infection.) Use only a sterile cleaning solution.

- For daily wear and rigid, gas-permeable lenses, use an additional protein-removing enzyme cleaner.
- With soft contacts, some bacteria can penetrate the lenses. After rubbing each lens in the palm of your hand for a few seconds, soak it in a cleaning solution for at least four hours before wearing it again. This should kill most of the remaining bacteria.
- Clean your lens case daily with the sterile rinsing solution and let it air-dry. Replace the case every three months.

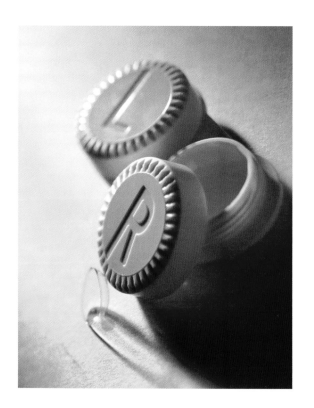

Refractive surgery

If you're tired of wearing eyeglasses or contact lenses, you may be among the millions of people considering an increasingly popular alternative — refractive surgery. Refractive surgery refers to surgical procedures that treat focusing problems of the eyes by correcting the curvature of the cornea. This type of surgery can correct far-sightedness, nearsightedness and astigmatism, though it can't help you with presbyopia — the decline in your reading vision that usually starts when you reach your 40s.

The popularity of refractive surgery is due partly to intensive marketing and partly to the surgery's effectiveness — it really does allow many people to get rid of their glasses or contacts. Refractive surgery may be especially attractive if you work in a dusty job and wear contacts, or if you're constantly going in and out of doors in cold weather and dealing with foggy glasses. When swimming or water-skiing, glasses or contact lenses can be impractical or impossible to wear.

LASIK eye surgery — short for laser-assisted in-situ keratomileusis — is the most common type of refractive surgery. With increasing experience and advances in technology, the outcomes and predictability of LASIK surgery have greatly improved in recent years. But complications associated with LASIK still exist, and the procedure usually isn't covered by insurance. Before you schedule this type of surgery, find out what it entails and what could go wrong.

Preparing for LASIK

For your eyes to focus light accurately, three elements must be precisely coordinated — the shape of the cornea, the condition of the natural lens and the length of the eyeball. In normally shaped eyeballs, the cornea and the lens bend light so that it focuses a sharp image directly on the light-sensitive retina at the back of the eye.

LASIK eye surgery improves vision by changing one of these elements — the curvature of the cornea. After the procedure, your cornea should bend light rays to adjust for any misalignment and focus the image more precisely on your retina.

A good surgical outcome depends on careful evaluation of your eyes before you turn to LASIK surgery or similar procedures. Your eye doctor may recommend that you first try other methods of correcting your vision, such as glasses or contact lenses.

Unlike sight-threatening eye diseases, refractive errors aren't progressive in themselves, and they may actually improve in middle age. Some doctors are reluctant to endorse LASIK, reasoning that your eyes are basically healthy even if you have nearsightedness or farsightedness.

Before refractive surgery, the surgeon typically gathers a detailed medical history and uses specialized equipment to carefully measure the cornea, noting its shape, thickness and any irregularities.

If you wear contact lenses, you'll need to switch to glasses full time for a few weeks before this exam. Contact lenses can distort the shape

Presbyopia and LASIK

Presbyopia refers to difficulty reading and seeing things close up that naturally comes with age (see page 163). It happens as the natural lens gradually loses its ability to change shape. For older adults with no other need for corrective lenses, the condition is usually well managed with reading glasses. For people seeking to avoid glasses, LASIK surgery may provide some benefits with certain limitations.

If you use LASIK surgery to correct your reading vision, the changes will likely cause you to need glasses or contacts for distance vision. (And correcting for distance vision will likely make your presbyopia worse!) To avoid this, you might choose to have your vision corrected for monovision. With monovision, one eye is corrected for distance vision and the other for reading vision. Not everyone is able to adjust to or tolerate monovision, so it's wise to undergo a trial with contact lenses before opting for a permanent surgical procedure.

of your cornea, which could lead to inaccurate measurements and a poor surgical outcome.

Skip eye makeup and eye cream on the days prior to your surgery. Your doctor may also instruct you to clean your eyelashes in the days leading up to surgery, to remove debris and minimize your risk of infection.

Refractive surgery is usually considered an elective surgery — which means it isn't vital to your health and well-being. For this reason, Medicare and most insurance companies don't cover the cost of the surgery.

The LASIK procedure

LASIK is performed using a laser that's programmed to remove a defined amount of tissue from your cornea. Often, surgery is performed on both eyes on the same day.

During the pre-surgical eye exam, your eye doctor uses highly specialized instruments to determine specific areas of your cornea that need to be flattened or curved. This allows your doctor to chart your eye and remove tissue from the cornea precisely. Wave front-guided LASIK, a new type of LASIK procedure, uses a special device called a wave front scanner that allows your doctor to create a highly detailed chart — like a topographical map — of your eye. Theoretically, the more detailed the measurements, the more accurately your doctor can remove corneal tissue to improve your vision.

Just prior to surgery, you'll receive anesthetic eyedrops that numb your eye during the procedure, which helps ensure you'll experience little pain. You may also be given medicine to help you relax.

During surgery. LASIK surgery usually takes less than 30 minutes. During the procedure, you'll lie on your back in a reclining chair. After the numbing drops are placed in your eye, your doctor uses a special instrument to hold your eyelids open. A suction ring is positioned on your eye, which may cause a feeling of pressure and your vision may dim a little.

As the procedure is taking place, you'll be asked to focus on a point of light. Staring at this light helps you keep your eye fixed while the laser reshapes your cornea.

The surgeon uses a delicate blade, called a microkeratome, or a cutting laser to cut a circular flap of tissue from the center of your cornea. This flap, still hinged to the cornea, is about the size and shape of a contact lens. The surgeon folds this flap out of the way and uses a laser to reshape the layers of the cornea underneath the flap — removing one microscopic layer at a time.

You may detect a distinct odor as the laser removes corneal tissue. Some people describe smelling an odor similar to burning hair. After the reshaping is complete, the flap is folded back into place and usually heals without stitches.

After surgery. You'll need to have someone drive you to and from your surgery. Immediately after surgery, your eyes may burn or itch and be watery. Your vision also may be blurry. You might still feel the effects of the medication given to you before surgery.

You may be given pain medication or eyedrops to keep you comfortable for several hours after the procedure.

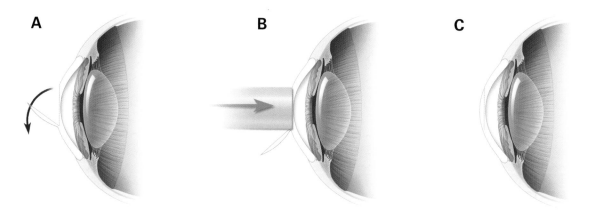

LASIK surgery

To begin the LASIK procedure, your surgeon uses a special blade or laser to cut a circular flap on the top layer of your cornea. Folding back this flap allows access to deeper layers of tissue (A). A laser reshapes the exposed tissue, making it flatter or steeper depending on your needs for corrected vision (B). When reshaping is complete, the corneal flap is repositioned over the treated area and allowed to heal on its own (C).

You may also need to wear a shield over your eye at night until it heals.

Typically, you're able to see after the procedure but your vision won't necessarily be better right away. Expect your vision to improve over the next two to three months. Most people who have refractive surgery eventually attain 20/25 vision or better. Your chances for improved vision are based, in part, on how good your vision was before surgery.

You'll likely see your doctor a day or two after surgery and at regular intervals for the next few months.

Who shouldn't have LASIK

LASIK surgery poses particular risks for some people. You should not have this surgery if you have:

- **Immune system disease.** Diseases that affect your immune system may impair your ability to heal after surgery. The risks of incomplete healing, infection and other complications are increased if you have an autoimmune disease, such as rheumatoid arthritis, or an immunodeficiency disease, such as HIV. Taking an immunosup-

pressive drug also disqualifies you from having this surgery.
- **Persistent dry eyes.** Any condition that causes dry eyes, including the disease Sjogren's syndrome, is likely to impair healing.
- **Certain eye characteristics.** An extremely uneven corneal surface or an otherwise abnormally shaped cornea may make surgery more difficult to perform.
- **Unstable vision.** If the quality of your vision fluctuates or is progressively worsening, you may not be eligible for LASIK surgery.
- **You're not an adult.** Currently, no lasers used in refractive surgery are approved for use on individuals under the age of 18.
- **Other factors.** For example, deep-set eyes or thin corneas may make the surgery more difficult.

Refractive surgery also may not be a good choice if:
- **It jeopardizes your career.** Some jobs, in which very precise vision is required, may prohibit certain refractive procedures.
- **Cost is an issue.** Although refractive surgery is becoming less expensive, it's still a significant cost and most insurance companies don't pay for the procedure.

- **You have high refractive error.** If you have severe nearsightedness — you have a strong prescription — the surgery may not be able to produce acceptable results.
- **You have low refractive error.** If your vision is pretty good and you only need to wear contacts or glasses some of the time, improvement from the surgery may not be worth the risk of complications.
- **You have large pupils.** Refractive surgery performed on individuals prone to having large pupils in dim light can result in debilitating symptoms such as glare, halos, star bursts and ghost images.
- **You actively participate in contact sports.** If you frequently partici-

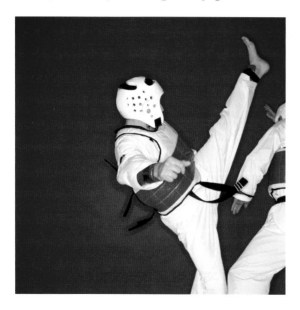

pate in boxing, martial arts or other activities in which blows to the face and eyes are a normal occurrence, refractive surgery may not be in your best interest.

Other refractive procedures

If you're not a good candidate for LASIK surgery, your eye doctor may recommend another type of refractive surgery. These include:

Photorefractive keratectomy. Photorefractive keratectomy (PRK) is better suited to some people while LASIK is to others. PRK is sometimes used if you have a low to moderate degree of nearsightedness or farsightedness, or if you have nearsightedness with astigmatism.

During PRK, your surgeon uses an excimer laser to remove the outermost surface of the cornea and re-sculpt the curvature of the cornea, making it slightly flatter. The excimer laser doesn't cut or burn tissue. It emits a "cold," or nonthermal, light beam and allows controlled amounts of tissue to be removed from the corneal surface, one microscopic layer at a time. PRK also doesn't involve creating a "flap" of tissue, which must be repositioned after the surgery. Most people have surgery on both eyes on the same day.

With PRK, the exposed surface of your cornea naturally repairs itself, often assisted by a temporary contact lens you wear as a "bandage" over your eye for three or four days after surgery. You may have eye pain for a few days until your cornea heals. It generally takes up to a week for your eye to regenerate the surface tissue that was removed. It may take three to six months before your vision improves completely.

In general, PRK is less commonly performed than LASIK. Healing after LASIK tends to be more predictable and usually involves less discomfort. However, thanks to improved technology, PRK is experiencing a bit of a rebound. With PRK, healing takes longer but there's generally less risk because there are no flap complications to worry about.

Laser epithelial keratomileusis (LASEK). LASEK is a similar to LASIK surgery. During LASEK surgery, a much thinner layer — the surface layer (epithelium) — of your cornea is folded back to allow the laser to focus on parts of your cornea that need reshaping. The epithelial flap is then replaced.

If you have very thin corneas, you might be a good candidate for LASEK because the procedure allows your doctor to remove less of your cornea. As with LASIK, LASEK surgery can be done on both eyes on the same day.

Bladeless LASIK. With this procedure, the surgeon creates a flap in the cornea using an ultrafast and precise laser. The laser replaces the surgical blade that is traditionally used in LASIK surgery.

Implantable lenses. Phakic intraocular lenses are implantable lenses that are surgically inserted into the eye to improve vision. The technology works by placing an implantable lens in front of the natural lens. One of its advantages is that it has the capability to correct high degrees of nearsightedness that cannot be corrected with other surgical procedures.

Intracorneal ring segments (ICRS). Intracorneal ring segments are used to treat mild nearsightedness. A small incision is made in the cornea, and two crescent-shaped plastic rings are placed on the cornea's outer edge. The rings help flatten the cornea so that light rays focus on the retina.

Possible risks

As with any surgery, refractive surgery carries risks, including:

- **Undercorrection.** If the laser removes too little tissue from your eye, you won't get the vision results you were hoping for. You may need another surgery to remove more tissue.
- **Overcorrection.** It's possible that the laser will remove too much tissue from your eye. Overcorrections can be more difficult to fix than undercorrections.
- **Astigmatism.** Astigmatism may result from uneven tissue removal. This may occur if your eye moves too much during surgery, and may require additional surgery.
- **Glare, halos and double vision.** After surgery you may notice glare, halos around bright lights or double vision. Sometimes these signs and symptoms can be treated with corticosteroid eyedrops. Other times, a second surgery is required.

- **Dry eyes.** As your eyes heal after surgery, they may feel unusually dry. You'll likely need to use eyedrops during this time.
- **Flap problems.** Folding back or removing the flap from your eye during surgery can cause complications, including infection, tearing and swelling. The flap may also grow back abnormally.

Results

The goal of refractive surgery is for you to achieve "functional vision," which refers to a person's ability to do most daily tasks without corrective lenses. More than 90 percent of people who've undergone refractive surgery no longer need to use their glasses or contact lenses on a regular basis. In some situations, however, such as driving at night, you may still need corrective lenses to achieve your best vision. It should also be mentioned that 5 percent to 20 percent of people who undergo laser vision correction need a second surgery (enhancement surgery) to correct lingering focusing difficulties.

Chapter 9

Living with low vision

Several chapters in this book have explained how various eye diseases are diagnosed and treated. Although prompt treatment can stop or minimize further damage to your eyes, it doesn't always recover vision lost in early stages of the disease. In some cases, this damage can be extensive. With glaucoma, for example, your peripheral vision may almost completely disappear before you realize that something is wrong.

Permanent loss of vision may prevent you from doing many everyday tasks or from participating in activities that you enjoy. For example, you may not be able to read books and newspapers or safely move around your house. Or your eyes may not be able to adjust to bright lights and glare as you drive.

Vision loss can stem from a single disease, such as macular degeneration or glaucoma, or it may be the cumulative result of several conditions, such as diabetes, high blood pressure and obesity. Vision loss can also result from serious eye injuries or birth defects. The effects may range from mild to severe.

When your vision is compromised, you may have what's known as low vision. This is generally defined as vision that's 20/70 or worse and that cannot be corrected with standard eyeglasses, contact lenses or surgery. However, having low vision involves more than the numbers from a visual acuity assessment. Your eye doctor also needs to determine how much the loss interferes with your everyday needs and activities. According to the National Eye Institute, low vision may cause:

- Problems doing close-up work, including reading, cooking, sewing and hobbies
- Problems differentiating colors, particularly those in the green, blue and violet hues
- Difficulty seeing because lights seem dimmer than they used to be

Defining low vision

There are different levels of low vision — from mild to more severe loss of sight. Low vision is often categorized as follows, based on the level of vision in the better eye:

Moderate low vision	20/70 to 20/160
Severe low vision	20/200 to 20/400
Profound low vision	20/500 to 20/1,000
Near-total vision loss	Vision worse than 20/1,000

There are other categories of visual impairment based on the loss of peripheral vision (visual field loss).

In the United States, any person with vision that cannot be corrected to better than 20/200 in the best eye, or who has 20 degrees or less of visual field remaining, is considered legally blind. Being legally blind, however, is not the same as total blindness. Unlike a person who is completely blind, a person with severe or profound low vision has some useful sight.

- Trouble reading street, bus or store signs
- Difficulty recognizing the faces of relatives and friends

Living with vision loss isn't an easy experience for anyone, but it's important to know that you can still meet many of your functional needs and live a relatively independent life. A variety of techniques and devices can help you make the most of your remaining vision.

Vision rehabilitation

Many people with low vision believe that there's little that can be done for them — that from here on out, life is a downhill path with diminishing rewards. The reality is, many types of vision loss respond well to vision rehabilitation, also known as low-vision rehabilitation.

What is vision rehabilitation? It's a combination of specialized training and counseling services that can help you develop special skills that allow you to continue taking part in day-to-

day activities. Vision rehabilitation cannot restore your vision, but it can give you self-assurance and allow you to maintain a greater degree of independence.

Vision rehabilitation starts with an assessment by a low-vision specialist. This person is an eye doctor trained in evaluating people with low vision. He or she may also work with other health care professionals, such as social workers, occupational therapists and others, to maximize your remaining vision.

A visit with a low-vision specialist generally begins with a complete history of your vision, during which you may be asked to describe tasks that you're having difficulty performing. The specialist will then decide on a course of testing. During testing, your knowledge of and comfort in using low-vision aids such as glasses, magnifiers, telescopes and electronic devices, as well as nonoptical devices such as reading stands, lamps and writing templates, is evaluated.

Testing is not just a trial-and-error process, although sometimes it may seem that way. Often testing must be done over several visits — as this process takes time — and can be fatiguing. A low-vision examination is carried out in a manner designed to maximize your vision and to achieve the goals set by you and the specialist at the start of testing.

Once a low-vision specialist determines the best aids for you, he or she may develop a training program that provides you with a thorough understanding of low-vision aids and their use. The program may be carried out by the specialist with his or her staff or by another professional, such as a vision rehabilitation specialist.

This training is important because as simple as these aids may seem, if they're not used properly, they won't function in the manner they're intended to. Just as someone who's experienced physical trauma or a stroke may need rehabilitation to relearn how to do simple tasks, people with low vision may need to learn to do daily activities in a slightly different way.

Rehabilitation for low vision generally involves three areas: independent living skills, orientation and mobility training, and use of assistive or adaptive technology.

Independent living skills

An integral part of vision rehabilitation therapy is relearning how to perform basic tasks. This covers a wide array of activities and adaptations, from using the telephone and writing checks, to improving lighting and making your home safer and more efficient to live in.

Several types of professionals — from vision rehabilitation specialists to occupational therapists — may assist you through this process.

Grooming and dressing

Feeling good about your appearance can help boost your self-esteem. The more confident you feel, the more determined you may be to overcome difficulties associated with low vision. Here are tips to help you look your best.
- Request a hairstyle that's easy to manage from your stylist or barber.
- Purchase shampoo, conditioner, body wash and other toiletries in bottles of different sizes and

shapes so that you can easily tell them apart.

- Learn to select and apply makeup from a rehabilitation specialist.
- Differentiate your favorite lipstick shades with rubber bands. For example, red has no band, pink has one band and coral has two bands around the container.
- Use dark-colored or striped toothpaste to contrast with the white bristles on your toothbrush, making it easier to get the paste on the brush.
- For shaving safety, try using an electric razor.
- To determine the color of your clothes, place a large label over each hanger with letters such as BR for brown, B for black and R for red on the label. You can also pin a label to the front of the item.
- Organize clothing into matching outfits. For example, place an ensemble of pants, shirt and tie on one hanger.

Cooking

There's no need for fear in the kitchen. A person with low vision can learn to cook just as well as a person with normal sight. It starts by honing your senses: Feel the vibration of the

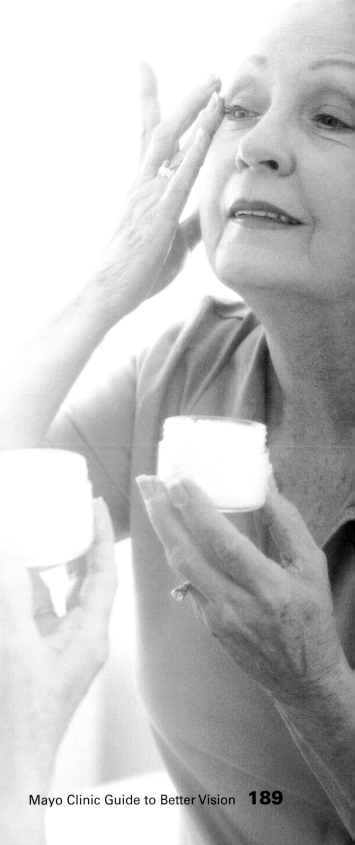

boiling water on the kettle handle. Hear the popping of frying food to know it's browning. Learn to smell when something is done. In addition:

- Always store utensils, pots and pans, spices and other cooking items in the same locations so that you can find them easily. Smell spices before you use them.
- Look for adaptive versions of common kitchen equipment, such as large-print measuring cups, kitchen timers with raised-print markings and long oven mitts that cover the arms.
- Organize food items in your pantry in a familiar manner. To help distinguish items, have a friend or family member mark the item in big letters with a dark, felt-tipped pen. You can also use the rubber band system, for example, no band for tomato soup, one band for vegetable soup and two bands for cream of mushroom.
- Install under-the-counter lighting at locations where you do food preparation.
- On appliance knobs and dials, file a small notch or apply bump dots or drops of glue or nail polish to frequently used settings. On your oven, you might mark every 100 degrees.

- Use a cutting board that contrasts with the color of the food item you're cutting.
- Look for helpful shortcuts. Consider using frozen vegetables instead of chopping fresh ones. Ask the butcher to cube a piece of beef for you.
- Use slow cookers, bread machines and other appliances that simplify the cooking process.

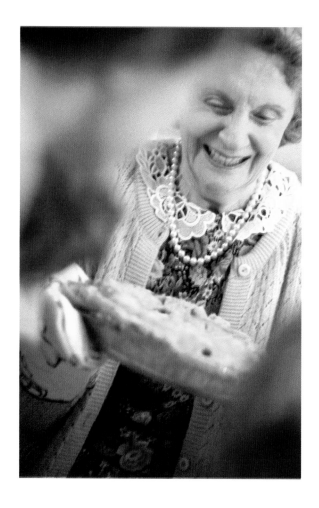

Using the telephone

Following are a few simple steps to make communicating on the telephone easier:

- Inquire with your phone company regarding services for customers with special needs. This may include large-print billing and large-print telephone books.
- Obtain a large-print number template to place on top of your existing telephone so that you can see the numbers more easily.
- Purchase a telephone with a memory system, which enables you to dial complete numbers by pressing just one button.
- Consider attaching a device to your telephone that allows you to pick up the receiver, say the name of the person you're planning to call, and the device dials the complete number for you.

Managing money

Identifying the correct values of coins and currency can be a problem if your vision is limited. Writing checks and paying bills also can be frustrating. Here are some tips that might help make managing your money a little easier:

- Fold paper currency in ways that help you determine which bills you have by feeling them with your fingers. For example, place $1 bills in your wallet flat and unfolded. Fold $5 bills lengthwise to make a long and thin rectangle. Fold $10 bills in half, making them square shaped. Fold $20 bills twice: first, long and thin like the $5 bill, and then in half, to make a small, thick rectangle.
- Coin identification is simple once you've studied the size, texture and thickness of each coin.
- When making a purchase, try to use a combination of bills and coins that's close to the amount of sale, minimizing how much change you'll receive. Ask the cashier to say aloud what bills you're receiving as change, so you'll know how to sort them.
- Find out if your bank offers large-print checks or checks printed with raised lines. Also ask about check guides. These are opaque templates with openings that indicate where you need to fill in information, such as the amount of purchase and your signature. Other options for money transactions include online banking and banking by phone.

- Inquire about a talking calculator, which announces which keys you've just pressed and reports the results.

Taking medications

Whether it's a daily vitamin or a prescription medication, many people take one or more pills on a daily basis. To help keep track of what you're taking, consider these tips:

- Use labels or markings to differentiate the different bottles. You might do this by color-coding the bottles or by printing large letters and numbers on their sides. You can also mark the covers with bump dots or drops of glue and nail polish.
- Request that your pharmacist use different-sized bottles to help differentiate your prescription medications.
- Learn to recognize each pill by its shape and size.
- Wrap rubber bands around the bottle equal to the number of daily doses. This will help you remember if you've taken the right amount. Another option is a pill organizer with a beeping alarm to alert you when it's time for the next dose.

Making a safe environment

Even in the comfortable surroundings of your home, it's important to take steps that make the environment safer. Here are a few suggestions:

- Arrange furniture so that sharp corners and edges don't obstruct your normal traffic patterns.
- Eliminate throw rugs and rearrange or secure other tripping hazards, such as loose extension cords. Keep the floor picked up of shoes, clothing, newspapers and other items.
- Raised door thresholds and steps can be difficult to see. Use safety tape or contrasting paint to highlight these areas, especially top and bottom steps. Make sure the stairways are well lit.
- Use sturdy banisters or grab rails on stairs and in the bathroom.
- Close closet doors and cupboard drawers as soon as you're done using them. Doors and drawers left partially open cause accidents.
- Install an intercom at your front door so that visitors can identify themselves.
- Install wireless sensor lights throughout the house so your pathway is always illuminated,

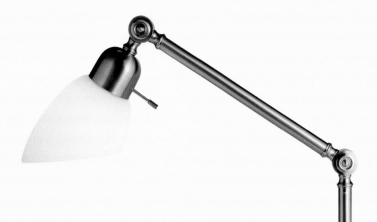

Lighting up your life

Even if you don't have a vision-limiting eye disorder, you'll need more light for close-up tasks as you get older. Good lighting also helps you avoid obstructions and trip hazards in your pathway.

Here are helpful lighting tips to remember if you're dealing with low vision:

- Minimize sharp contrasts by keeping the house lights on during the day to help equalize indoor and outdoor light sources. When reading or doing detail work, don't face the windows. Position yourself so that the windows are behind you or to the side.
- Use an adjustable lamp for reading or doing other close-up work. Two of the best options are a gooseneck lamp or a lamp with a swivel arm that can be raised or lowered. Position the lamp about four to eight inches from your reading material, but slightly off to the side to reduce glare.
- Direct your light source over the shoulder of the eye that has your best vision.
- Install lighting under shelves and cupboards in kitchen, study or work areas to increase visibility.
- Wear a visor or hat with a wide brim indoors to block annoying overhead light.

Many older adults experience increased sensitivity to glare caused by reflected sunlight or from other lighting sources. Polarized glass will help eliminate glare. If possible, choose furnishings with a flat or matte finish. Cover shiny surfaces, such as a polished table, with a cloth. Place a dark piece of construction paper behind your reading material to reduce glare when you read.

especially when you return home in the evening. A less expensive option is putting an automatic night light in your entry area.

- Mark the "start" position on the dials of your washing machine and dishwasher. Also mark the thermostat at a comfortable temperature setting. Consider installing a large-print or talking thermostat that gives you greater control of the home environment.
- Store similarly shaped containers, such as spray cans of insect repellent and air freshener, in separate locations. If possible, label or mark each container to help identify it.

Orientation and mobility training

It's not uncommon for individuals with low vision to be reluctant to travel outside of their homes, due to safety concerns and fear of getting lost. But the loss of independence — making it difficult to meet medical appointments or run to the grocery store — has a very negative impact on quality of life. Another key component of vision rehabilitation therapy is helping individuals with low vision feel more secure and confident outside their homes.

Orientation and mobility training may involve learning how to utilize any of the following: your remaining vision, the assistance of another person (sighted guide), a white cane or a guide dog. Training may be provided by a certified orientation and mobility specialist or by an individual with experience in helping people with visual impairment move about and travel.

Remaining vision

To travel safely relying on your own eyesight, your vision needs to be good enough to react to people and vehicles moving about you, as well as to see the dangers posed by curbs, stairs, posts, holes and other obstacles in your pathway. A certified orientation specialist can teach you specific techniques for moving about safely, making it possible for you to walk about your neighborhood or catch a bus to more distant locations.

For moving about within a more limited area — such as your backyard

— a few simple steps can help improve safety.

- Line all walkways with plants that differ sharply from the color of the walkway.
- Place low-voltage lighting along paths to help illuminate the walkway, especially on cloudy days or in the late afternoon and evening.
- Mark the edges of outdoor steps with paint or duct tape in a contrasting color.
- Remove anything from the yard that you could potentially trip over or run into, such as a clothesline.
- Always cross the street at the crosswalk, even if it's to a neighbor's house.

Sighted guide

If you're traveling beyond familiar surroundings, you may find it easier to rely on another person — a sighted guide — to help you get around. When walking with a sighted guide, still pay attention to your surroundings and look or listen for cues that help orient you. The guide will walk about half a step in front of you, and it's generally best to hold his or her arm just above the elbow. That way, you're better able to feel and follow the person's movements.

White cane

A white cane is used to detect obstacles in front of you, such as steps, curbs and uneven pavement. The color of the cane alerts passers-by to use caution and to not walk in front of you.

Canes come in different styles, including those that can be folded to fit into a coat pocket or purse. Although white canes can be ordered through catalogs, it's best to be "fitted" for a cane and to receive instruction on its use from an orientation and mobility specialist. When sizing a cane, you want it to be long enough

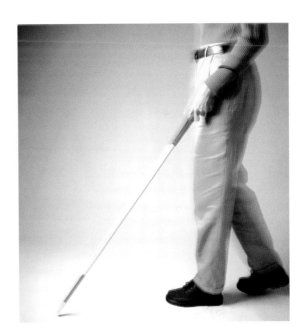

to give you sufficient reaction time and distance to prevent an injury, but not too long so that the cane is clumsy and difficult to use. As a rule of thumb, the cane should extend from the middle of your chest to the floor, and possibly a little longer.

Guide dog

Similar to a sighted guide, a guide dog can be your surrogate eyes — surveying the environment, leading you around obstacles and warning you of potential hazards. Many people with limited vision find a guide dog to be a great asset as well as a wonderful companion. However, it's important that you care for the dog properly and that you be willing to maintain his or her training.

Latest technology

A wide array of devices — everything from magnifying lenses and enlarged telephone dials to closed-circuit televisions and machines that talk — is available to help people with low vision remain actively involved in daily life. A low-vision specialist can help you find a device, or perhaps several devices, tailored to your specific vision problem. The devices are generally affordable and easy to use.

Assistive devices

Assistive devices are designed to help you use your remaining vision more effectively. They're frequently used in

Avoiding bumps in the road

Researchers continue to find new ways for technology to assist people with low vision. A device that can help people outside the home is called an electronic travel aid (ETA). Electronic travel aids help detect objects in your walking path by way of sonar or laser detection. If an object is detected, you'll receive a warning signal, such as a sound or vibration. Most often, ETAs are used in conjunction with a white cane or guide dog — providing extra protection and bolstering confidence.

conjunction with regular prescription glasses. Assistive devices include magnifiers for close-up work and telescopes for distance vision.

Magnifying eyeglasses. Magnifying eyeglasses contain a lens that's stronger than regular prescription eyeglasses. The magnifying lens can be mounted on your eyeglass frames or a special headband. This frees both of your hands for other tasks, such as holding a book comfortably. For the best vision, it's always important to have plenty of light.

Hand-held and stand magnifiers. Hand-held and stand magnifiers allow you to read print or work with objects positioned at a normal distance from your eyes. A hand-held magnifier may be carried with you for reading price tags, labels and restaurant menus. The device is less practical for activities such as continuous reading because you have to hold the lens at a steady distance from the reading material, which can be exhausting to your arms.

Stand magnifiers can be adjusted at a fixed distance directly above the object that you're looking at, such as a book. A low-vision specialist can help you choose the right type of magnifier with the correct power to assist with your particular vision problem.

Telescopes. Conventional magnifying lenses are intended for close-up work. They don't help you see better at a distance — even objects that are just across the room. A telescope magnifies objects in the distance, but at the expense of a greatly narrowed field of vision.

Telescopes may be held in the hand or mounted on eyeglasses. Hand-held telescopes are best used for short-term viewing, such as reading bus numbers and street signs. An eyeglass-mounted system is better for long-term viewing, for example, when you're watching television, an outdoor sporting event or a concert.

Many telescopes can be focused manually. Autofocus telescopes adjust focus automatically as the user changes the direction of his or her gaze, such as from a far-distance to intermediate-distance object.

Adaptive devices

Adaptive technology is the term used to describe devices — such as televisions and computers — that can be adapted to suit the needs of people who otherwise may not be able to use them. Adaptive devices generally fall into three broad categories — devices that make images or print bigger, devices that convert printed text to speech, and devices that display information in braille.

Screen magnifiers. Various magnifying devices and computer programs may function in different ways but have one goal in mind — to enlarge images and printed text on a screen.

A video magnifier — also referred to as a closed-circuit television system — provides much greater magnification than do standard optical devices. This device uses a video camera to project a magnified image onto a stand-alone screen, television screen or computer monitor. Video magnifiers help people with low vision read books and newspapers, manage their checkbooks, or look at photos.

There are video magnifiers with different capabilities, depending on what suits your needs. With the basic, fixed model, you pass the material you want to read or look at under the camera. The camera magnifies the object and displays it on the monitor.

Hand-held or head-mounted systems are designed for bringing the camera closer to the object that you want to view. You can also purchase video magnifiers that connect to your computer, allowing you to adjust the magnification to a size that works best for you. You can adjust the color, brightness, contrast and background of the screen to suit your needs.

In addition to video magnifiers, you can purchase specialized computer software programs that magnify all text that appears on your computer screen, making it easier for you to read documents, e-mail and information that you find on the Internet. Some programs may have expanded capabilities to help make it easier to use the computer.

Speech systems. Individuals with severe vision impairment often resort to speech systems. Instead of magnifying text on a monitor screen, these special devices scan text and read it aloud to you.

There are two main types of speech systems. With one type, printed text is placed under a scanning device, similar to a video magnifier. An internal camera scans the print and then reads it aloud with a synthetic voice. The device can read almost anything that's printed, but it doesn't work with handwritten material. You can use this type of speech system by itself or you can connect it to your computer. When it's linked to a computer, the scanned material can be converted into other forms, such as braille or large print.

Another type of speech system involves a synthetic voice device or program installed on your computer. The synthesizer reads aloud the text on your computer monitor. It also tells you what actions are taking place on screen: where the cursor is, what text is highlighted and other essential computer activities.

Braille technology. The braille writing system is based on patterns of raised dots arranged in cells, or small rectangles, of up to six dots. Adaptive technology that uses braille includes displays, printers and note takers.

Braille displays allow people with low vision to read the information on a computer screen. The devices work by electronically raising and lowering different combinations of pins, which

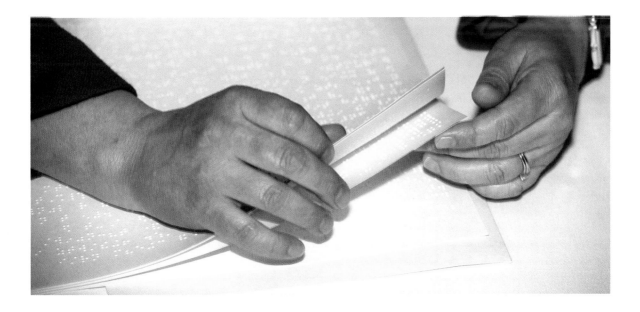

you feel with your fingertips. The pins change as the user moves the cursor around the computer screen. Braille printers work like other computer printers only the information is printed in braille. Note takers equipped for braille are small, portable devices for entering information using a braille keyboard. The devices output information by way of either a speech synthesizer or a braille display. You can transfer this information from the note taker to your personal computer.

Talking devices

Everyone loves a good gadget, and some of these gadgets can be very helpful to people with low vision. You may be surprised at the variety of everyday items that can be equipped with a synthetic voice. Here are a few of the items that can talk to you:

- Clocks
- Watches
- Timers
- Prescription bottles and medication reminders
- Bathroom scales
- Thermometers for taking your temperature
- Blood pressure monitors and glucose meters
- Calculators
- Indoor and outdoor thermometers
- Books and magazines

Index